Managing Common
Interventional Radiology
Complications

Lakshmi Ratnam • Uday Patel
Anna Maria Belli
Editors

Managing Common Interventional Radiology Complications

A Case Based Approach

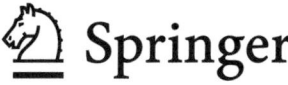 Springer

Editors
Lakshmi Ratnam
Department of Radiology
St. George's Hospital
London
UK

Anna Maria Belli
Department of Radiology
St. George's Hospital
London
UK

Uday Patel
Department of Radiology
St. George's Hospital
and Medical School
London
UK

ISBN 978-1-4471-5501-0   ISBN 978-1-4471-5502-7   (eBook)
DOI 10.1007/978-1-4471-5502-7
Springer London Heidelberg New York Dordrecht

Library of Congress Control Number: 2013954803

© Springer-Verlag London 2014
This work is subject to copyright. All rights are reserved by the Publisher, whether the whole or part of the material is concerned, specifically the rights of translation, reprinting, reuse of illustrations, recitation, broadcasting, reproduction on microfilms or in any other physical way, and transmission or information storage and retrieval, electronic adaptation, computer software, or by similar or dissimilar methodology now known or hereafter developed. Exempted from this legal reservation are brief excerpts in connection with reviews or scholarly analysis or material supplied specifically for the purpose of being entered and executed on a computer system, for exclusive use by the purchaser of the work. Duplication of this publication or parts thereof is permitted only under the provisions of the Copyright Law of the Publisher's location, in its current version, and permission for use must always be obtained from Springer. Permissions for use may be obtained through RightsLink at the Copyright Clearance Center. Violations are liable to prosecution under the respective Copyright Law.
The use of general descriptive names, registered names, trademarks, service marks, etc. in this publication does not imply, even in the absence of a specific statement, that such names are exempt from the relevant protective laws and regulations and therefore free for general use.
While the advice and information in this book are believed to be true and accurate at the date of publication, neither the authors nor the editors nor the publisher can accept any legal responsibility for any errors or omissions that may be made. The publisher makes no warranty, express or implied, with respect to the material contained herein.

Printed on acid-free paper

Springer is part of Springer Science+Business Media (www.springer.com)

To all our teachers

Preface

Although among the younger medical specialities, interventional radiology has rapidly established a central position in modern medical practice. The number and range of IR procedures is now wide and new procedures are pioneered all the time.

Whether of a minor nature – say, image guided biopsy or drainage – or complex, such as superselective arterial embolization and EVAR, IR techniques have a high success rate, but more importantly being minimally invasive the morbidity is more favourable compared to alternative procedures, be they surgical or medical. Nevertheless, complications can and do occur, and it is the duty of every IR practitioner to not only understand how and why such complications occur, so that they can be avoided, but also be technically armed to rectify the complication as speedily and safely as possible. Although any complication is in its way unique, there are always common themes.

An anonymized format has been adopted, by listing all the contributors to this book jointly at the head of each chapter describing a real complication. The practitioners who dealt with the complication describe how they managed the problem and the eventual outcome. Each chapter also discusses how such problems arise and the principles behind their early recognition and eventual management. Some general tips are also given for the benefit of those who have not yet encountered such a complication.

Finally, a general commentary is provided, written by the editors, which is a reflection on the problem and describes, when applicable, alternative strategies to the complication.

London, UK	Dr. Lakshmi Ratnam
London, UK	Dr. Uday Patel
London, UK	Prof. Anna Maria Belli

Acknowledgements

The editors are deeply grateful to all the authors who shared their clinical experience, without whom this book would have not been feasible. The help and encouragement of our IR colleagues and staff is also gratefully acknowledged. Finally, we would like to say thank you to our family and friends for always being there.

Contents

1 **Embolization Coil Trapped in the Side Hole of a Catheter**.............................. 1
Robert P. Allison, Anna Maria Belli,
Joo-Young Chun, Raymond Chung, Raj Das,
Andrew England, Karen Flood,
Marie-France Giroux, Richard G. McWilliams,
Robert Morgan, Nik Papadakos, Jai V. Patel,
Raf Patel, Uday Patel, Lakshmi Ratnam,
Reddi Prasad Yadavali, and John Rose

2 **Retrieval of an Intravascular Foreign Body in the Venous System**.................... 7
Robert P. Allison, Anna Maria Belli,
Joo-Young Chun, Raymond Chung, Raj Das,
Andrew England, Karen Flood,
Marie-France Giroux, Richard G. McWilliams,
Robert Morgan, Nik Papadakos, Jai V. Patel,
Raf Patel, Uday Patel, Lakshmi Ratnam,
Reddi Prasad Yadavali, and John Rose

3 **Migrated Superior Vena Cava Stent Repositioned Using a Balloon and Loop Snare Combination**................. 13
Robert P. Allison, Anna Maria Belli,
Joo-Young Chun, Raymond Chung, Raj Das,
Andrew England, Karen Flood,
Marie-France Giroux, Richard G. McWilliams,
Robert Morgan, Nik Papadakos, Jai V. Patel,
Raf Patel, Uday Patel, Lakshmi Ratnam,
Reddi Prasad Yadavali, and John Rose

4 **Retrieval of Central Venous Catheter Fragment
   Following Portacath Removal** 21
   Robert P. Allison, Anna Maria Belli,
   Joo-Young Chun, Raymond Chung, Raj Das,
   Andrew England, Karen Flood,
   Marie-France Giroux, Richard G. McWilliams,
   Robert Morgan, Nik Papadakos, Jai V. Patel,
   Raf Patel, Uday Patel, Lakshmi Ratnam,
   Reddi Prasad Yadavali, and John Rose

5 **Central Venous Catheter Inserted
   into the Mediastinum** 29
   Robert P. Allison, Anna Maria Belli,
   Joo-Young Chun, Raymond Chung, Raj Das,
   Andrew England, Karen Flood,
   Marie-France Giroux, Richard G. McWilliams,
   Robert Morgan, Nik Papadakos, Jai V. Patel,
   Raf Patel, Uday Patel, Lakshmi Ratnam,
   Reddi Prasad Yadavali, and John Rose

6 **Femoral Artery Pseudoaneurysm Treated
   with Percutaneous Thrombin Injection** 37
   Robert P. Allison, Anna Maria Belli,
   Joo-Young Chun, Raymond Chung, Raj Das,
   Andrew England, Karen Flood,
   Marie-France Giroux, Richard G. McWilliams,
   Robert Morgan, Nik Papadakos, Jai V. Patel,
   Raf Patel, Uday Patel, Lakshmi Ratnam,
   Reddi Prasad Yadavali, and John Rose

7 **Superficial Femoral Artery Thrombosis
   Post-angioplasty** 45
   Robert P. Allison, Anna Maria Belli,
   Joo-Young Chun, Raymond Chung, Raj Das,
   Andrew England, Karen Flood,
   Marie-France Giroux, Richard G. McWilliams,
   Robert Morgan, Nik Papadakos, Jai V. Patel,
   Raf Patel, Uday Patel, Lakshmi Ratnam,
   Reddi Prasad Yadavali, and John Rose

**8 Superficial Femoral
Artery Rupture Following Angioplasty** 55
Robert P. Allison, Anna Maria Belli,
Joo-Young Chun, Raymond Chung, Raj Das,
Andrew England, Karen Flood,
Marie-France Giroux, Richard G. McWilliams,
Robert Morgan, Nik Papadakos, Jai V. Patel,
Raf Patel, Uday Patel, Lakshmi Ratnam,
Reddi Prasad Yadavali, and John Rose

**9 Distal Embolization Following Common Iliac
and Superficial Femoral Artery Angioplasty** 63
Robert P. Allison, Anna Maria Belli,
Joo-Young Chun, Raymond Chung, Raj Das,
Andrew England, Karen Flood,
Marie-France Giroux, Richard G. McWilliams,
Robert Morgan, Nik Papadakos, Jai V. Patel,
Raf Patel, Uday Patel, Lakshmi Ratnam,
Reddi Prasad Yadavali, and John Rose

**10 Flow-Limiting Iliac Artery Dissection
Post-angioplasty** 69
Robert P. Allison, Anna Maria Belli,
Joo-Young Chun, Raymond Chung, Raj Das,
Andrew England, Karen Flood,
Marie-France Giroux, Richard G. McWilliams,
Robert Morgan, Nik Papadakos, Jai V. Patel,
Raf Patel, Uday Patel, Lakshmi Ratnam,
Reddi Prasad Yadavali, and John Rose

**11 Dissection of Superior Mesenteric Artery
(SMA) During Transarterial Chemoembolization
(TACE) via a Replaced Right Hepatic Artery** 75
Robert P. Allison, Anna Maria Belli,
Joo-Young Chun, Raymond Chung, Raj Das,
Andrew England, Karen Flood,
Marie-France Giroux, Richard G. McWilliams,
Robert Morgan, Nik Papadakos, Jai V. Patel,
Raf Patel, Uday Patel, Lakshmi Ratnam,
Reddi Prasad Yadavali, and John Rose

12 Iatrogenic Iliac Artery Rupture During Arterial Stenting 83
Robert P. Allison, Anna Maria Belli,
Joo-Young Chun, Raymond Chung, Raj Das,
Andrew England, Karen Flood,
Marie-France Giroux, Richard G. McWilliams,
Robert Morgan, Nik Papadakos, Jai V. Patel,
Raf Patel, Uday Patel, Lakshmi Ratnam,
Reddi Prasad Yadavali, and John Rose

13 Detachment of a Balloon-Expandable Stent from the Balloon and the Wire 89
Robert P. Allison, Anna Maria Belli,
Joo-Young Chun, Raymond Chung, Raj Das,
Andrew England, Karen Flood,
Marie-France Giroux, Richard G. McWilliams,
Robert Morgan, Nik Papadakos, Jai V. Patel,
Raf Patel, Uday Patel, Lakshmi Ratnam,
Reddi Prasad Yadavali, and John Rose

14 Migration of Common Hepatic Artery Stent Graft Occluding Right Hepatic Artery Flow 97
Robert P. Allison, Anna Maria Belli,
Joo-Young Chun, Raymond Chung, Raj Das,
Andrew England, Karen Flood,
Marie-France Giroux, Richard G. McWilliams,
Robert Morgan, Nik Papadakos, Jai V. Patel,
Raf Patel, Uday Patel, Lakshmi Ratnam,
Reddi Prasad Yadavali, and John Rose

15 Migrated Stent Graft During TIPS Revision 105
Robert P. Allison, Anna Maria Belli,
Joo-Young Chun, Raymond Chung, Raj Das,
Andrew England, Karen Flood,
Marie-France Giroux, Richard G. McWilliams,
Robert Morgan, Nik Papadakos, Jai V. Patel,
Raf Patel, Uday Patel, Lakshmi Ratnam,
Reddi Prasad Yadavali, and John Rose

16	**Type 1A Endoleak Following EVAR Treated with a Proximal Cuff**...............	113

Robert P. Allison, Anna Maria Belli,
Joo-Young Chun, Raymond Chung, Raj Das,
Andrew England, Karen Flood,
Marie-France Giroux, Richard G. McWilliams,
Robert Morgan, Nik Papadakos, Jai V. Patel,
Raf Patel, Uday Patel, Lakshmi Ratnam,
Reddi Prasad Yadavali, and John Rose

17	**Management of a Type 1B Endoleak Following EVAR**............................	121

Robert P. Allison, Anna Maria Belli,
Joo-Young Chun, Raymond Chung, Raj Das,
Andrew England, Karen Flood,
Marie-France Giroux, Richard G. McWilliams,
Robert Morgan, Nik Papadakos, Jai V. Patel,
Raf Patel, Uday Patel, Lakshmi Ratnam,
Reddi Prasad Yadavali, and John Rose

18	**Persistent Type 2 Endoleak Post-EVAR with Aneurysm Expansion**...................	129

Robert P. Allison, Anna Maria Belli,
Joo-Young Chun, Raymond Chung, Raj Das,
Andrew England, Karen Flood,
Marie-France Giroux, Richard G. McWilliams,
Robert Morgan, Nik Papadakos, Jai V. Patel,
Raf Patel, Uday Patel, Lakshmi Ratnam,
Reddi Prasad Yadavali, and John Rose

19	**Acute Renal Artery Occlusion and Trapped Renal Artery Catheter During Infrarenal AAA Stent Grafting**........................	139

Robert P. Allison, Anna Maria Belli,
Joo-Young Chun, Raymond Chung, Raj Das,
Andrew England, Karen Flood,
Marie-France Giroux, Richard G. McWilliams,
Robert Morgan, Nik Papadakos, Jai V. Patel,
Raf Patel, Uday Patel, Lakshmi Ratnam,
Reddi Prasad Yadavali, and John Rose

20 Maldeployment of the Contralateral Limb During EVAR 149
Robert P. Allison, Anna Maria Belli,
Joo-Young Chun, Raymond Chung, Raj Das,
Andrew England, Karen Flood,
Marie-France Giroux, Richard G. McWilliams,
Robert Morgan, Nik Papadakos, Jai V. Patel,
Raf Patel, Uday Patel, Lakshmi Ratnam,
Reddi Prasad Yadavali, and John Rose

21 Branch Endograft Disconnection and Impending Type 3 Endoleak Post-EVAR 157
Robert P. Allison, Anna Maria Belli,
Joo-Young Chun, Raymond Chung, Raj Das,
Andrew England, Karen Flood,
Marie-France Giroux, Richard G. McWilliams,
Robert Morgan, Nik Papadakos, Jai V. Patel,
Raf Patel, Uday Patel, Lakshmi Ratnam,
Reddi Prasad Yadavali, and John Rose

22 Hemorrhage Following Percutaneous Nephrostomy 167
Robert P. Allison, Anna Maria Belli,
Joo-Young Chun, Raymond Chung, Raj Das,
Andrew England, Karen Flood,
Marie-France Giroux, Richard G. McWilliams,
Robert Morgan, Nik Papadakos, Jai V. Patel,
Raf Patel, Uday Patel, Lakshmi Ratnam,
Reddi Prasad Yadavali, and John Rose

23 Injury to Bowel Following Transplant Nephrostomy Insertion 175
Robert P. Allison, Anna Maria Belli,
Joo-Young Chun, Raymond Chung, Raj Das,
Andrew England, Karen Flood,
Marie-France Giroux, Richard G. McWilliams,
Robert Morgan, Nik Papadakos, Jai V. Patel,
Raf Patel, Uday Patel, Lakshmi Ratnam,
Reddi Prasad Yadavali, and John Rose

24	**Renal Arterial Hemorrhage Following Renal Artery Stenting**..................... 183
	Robert P. Allison, Anna Maria Belli, Joo-Young Chun, Raymond Chung, Raj Das, Andrew England, Karen Flood, Marie-France Giroux, Richard G. McWilliams, Robert Morgan, Nik Papadakos, Jai V. Patel, Raf Patel, Uday Patel, Lakshmi Ratnam, Reddi Prasad Yadavali, and John Rose
25	**Pyrexia After Tumor Embolization: Infection Versus Post-embolization Syndrome**............. 191
	Robert P. Allison, Anna Maria Belli, Joo-Young Chun, Raymond Chung, Raj Das, Andrew England, Karen Flood, Marie-France Giroux, Richard G. McWilliams, Robert Morgan, Nik Papadakos, Jai V. Patel, Raf Patel, Uday Patel, Lakshmi Ratnam, Reddi Prasad Yadavali, and John Rose
26	**Arterioportal Fistula and Liver Hemorrhage After Radiofrequency Ablation and TACE**....... 199
	Robert P. Allison, Anna Maria Belli, Joo-Young Chun, Raymond Chung, Raj Das, Andrew England, Karen Flood, Marie-France Giroux, Richard G. McWilliams, Robert Morgan, Nik Papadakos, Jai V. Patel, Raf Patel, Uday Patel, Lakshmi Ratnam, Reddi Prasad Yadavali, and John Rose
27	**Protrusion of Vena Cava Filter into the Aorta**............................. 205
	Robert P. Allison, Anna Maria Belli, Joo-Young Chun, Raymond Chung, Raj Das, Andrew England, Karen Flood, Marie-France Giroux, Richard G. McWilliams, Robert Morgan, Nik Papadakos, Jai V. Patel, Raf Patel, Uday Patel, Lakshmi Ratnam, Reddi Prasad Yadavali, and John Rose

28 The Multiple Options for Retrieval of a Tilted IVC Filter 213
Robert P. Allison, Anna Maria Belli,
Joo-Young Chun, Raymond Chung, Raj Das,
Andrew England, Karen Flood,
Marie-France Giroux, Richard G. McWilliams,
Robert Morgan, Nik Papadakos, Jai V. Patel,
Raf Patel, Uday Patel, Lakshmi Ratnam,
Reddi Prasad Yadavali, and John Rose

29 Retrieval of a Well-Orientated IVC Filter with Embedded Struts 221
Robert P. Allison, Anna Maria Belli,
Joo-Young Chun, Raymond Chung, Raj Das,
Andrew England, Karen Flood,
Marie-France Giroux, Richard G. McWilliams,
Robert Morgan, Nik Papadakos, Jai V. Patel,
Raf Patel, Uday Patel, Lakshmi Ratnam,
Reddi Prasad Yadavali, and John Rose

30 Retrieving a Tilted IVC Filter with Struts Penetrating the IVC 227
Robert P. Allison, Anna Maria Belli,
Joo-Young Chun, Raymond Chung, Raj Das,
Andrew England, Karen Flood,
Marie-France Giroux, Richard G. McWilliams,
Robert Morgan, Nik Papadakos, Jai V. Patel,
Raf Patel, Uday Patel, Lakshmi Ratnam,
Reddi Prasad Yadavali, and John Rose

31 Fistula Rupture Post-fistuloplasty 235
Robert P. Allison, Anna Maria Belli,
Joo-Young Chun, Raymond Chung, Raj Das,
Andrew England, Karen Flood,
Marie-France Giroux, Richard G. McWilliams,
Robert Morgan, Nik Papadakos, Jai V. Patel,
Raf Patel, Uday Patel, Lakshmi Ratnam,
Reddi Prasad Yadavali, and John Rose

**32 Circumferential Balloon Rupture
and Retained Fragments During Fistuloplasty
and Thrombolysis of a Thrombosed Fistula**....... 243
Robert P. Allison, Anna Maria Belli,
Joo-Young Chun, Raymond Chung, Raj Das,
Andrew England, Karen Flood,
Marie-France Giroux, Richard G. McWilliams,
Robert Morgan, Nik Papadakos, Jai V. Patel,
Raf Patel, Uday Patel, Lakshmi Ratnam,
Reddi Prasad Yadavali, and John Rose

**33 Hemorrhage After Transjugular
Liver Biopsy**................................. 251
Robert P. Allison, Anna Maria Belli,
Joo-Young Chun, Raymond Chung, Raj Das,
Andrew England, Karen Flood,
Marie-France Giroux, Richard G. McWilliams,
Robert Morgan, Nik Papadakos, Jai V. Patel,
Raf Patel, Uday Patel, Lakshmi Ratnam,
Reddi Prasad Yadavali, and John Rose

Index 259

Contributors

Robert P. Allison Department of Interventional Radiology, University Hospitals Southampton, Southampton, UK

Anna Maria Belli Department of Radiology, St. George's Hospital and Medical School, London, UK

Joo-Young Chun Department of Radiology, St. George's Hospital, London, UK

Raymond Chung Department of Radiology, St. George's Hospital, London, UK

Raj Das Department of Radiology, St. George's Hospital, London, UK

Andrew England Department of Radiography, University of Salford, Manchester, UK

Karen Flood Department of Vascular Radiology, Leeds General Infirmary, Leeds, UK

Marie-France Giroux Department of Radiology, CHUM-Centre Hospitalier de l'Université de Montréal, Montreal, QC, Canada

Richard G. McWilliams Department of Radiology, Royal Liverpool University Hospital, Liverpool, UK

Robert Morgan Department of Radiology, St. George's Hospital, London, UK

Nik Papadakos Department of Radiology, St. George's Hospital, London, UK

Jai V. Patel Department of Radiology, The Leeds Teaching Hospitals NHS Trust, Leeds, UK

Raf Patel Department of Radiology, The Leeds Teaching Hospitals NHS Trust, Leeds, West Yorkshire, UK

Uday Patel Department of Radiology, St. George's Hospital and Medical School, London, UK

Lakshmi Ratnam Department of Radiology, St. George's Hospital, London, UK

John Rose Department of Interventional Radiology, Freeman Hospital, Newcastle Upon Tyne Hospitals NHS Trust, Newcastle upon Tyne, UK

Reddi Prasad Yadavali Department of Radiology, Aberdeen Royal Infirmary, Aberdeen, UK

Chapter 1
Embolization Coil Trapped in the Side Hole of a Catheter

Robert P. Allison, Anna Maria Belli, Joo-Young Chun, Raymond Chung, Raj Das, Andrew England, Karen Flood, Marie-France Giroux, Richard G. McWilliams, Robert Morgan, Nik Papadakos, Jai V. Patel, Raf Patel, Uday Patel, Lakshmi Ratnam, Reddi Prasad Yadavali, and John Rose

Abstract This case illustrates the basic technique of retrieval of a displaced embolization coil. Catheter selection to avoid such a complication is discussed.

Keywords Embolization • Complications • Displaced coil • Coil retrieval

---

R.P. Allison
Department of Interventional Radiology,
University Hospitals Southampton, Southampton,
Hampshire, UK

A.M. Belli
Department of Radiology, St. George's Hospital
and Medical School, Blackshaw Road,
London SW17 0RE, UK
e-mail: anna.belli@stgeorges.nhs.uk

J.-Y. Chun • R. Chung • R. Das
R. Morgan • N. Papadakos
Department of Radiology, St. George's Hospital,
London, UK

A. England
Department of Radiography, University of Salford,
Manchester, UK

K. Flood
Department of Vascular Radiology, Leeds General
Infirmary, Leeds, UK

M.-F. Giroux
Department of Radiology, CHUM-Centre Hospitalier
de l'Université de Montréal, Montreal, QC, Canada

R.G. McWilliams
Department of Radiology, Royal Liverpool
University Hospital, Liverpool, UK

J.V. Patel
Department of Radiology, The Leeds Teaching
Hospitals NHS Trust, Leeds, West Yorkshire, UK

R. Patel
Department of Radiology,
The Leeds Teaching Hospitals NHS Trust,
Leeds, West Yorkshire, UK
e-mail: rafpatel@gmail.com

U. Patel
Department of Radiology,
St. George's Hospital and Medical School,
Blackshaw Road, SW17 0QT London, UK
e-mail: uday.patel@stgeorges.nhs.uk

L. Ratnam
Department of Radiology, St. George's Hospital,
Blackshaw Road, SW17 0QT London, UK
e-mail: lakshmi.ratnam@nhs.net

R.P. Yadavali
Department of Radiology, Aberdeen Royal Infirmary,
Aberdeen, UK

J. Rose
Department of Interventional Radiology,
Freeman Hospital, Newcastle Upon Tyne
Hospitals NHS Trust, Newcastle upon Tyne, UK

Chapter 1. Embolization coil trapped in catheter side hole

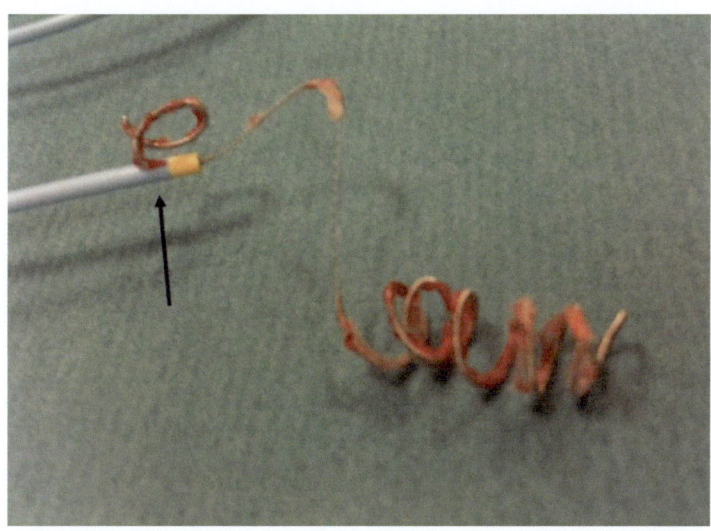

FIGURE 1.1 Coil protruding through the catheter side hole (*arrow*) and stretched by the retrieval attempts

Case History

A 28-year-old man with a symptomatic left-sided varicocele was referred to Interventional Radiology for embolization. He was otherwise fit and well. Ultrasound (US) examination of the scrotum revealed normal testes with a left-sided varicocele.

Procedure

A 6 Fr sheath was placed in the right internal jugular vein using US guidance. The left gonadal vein was catheterized without difficulty using a multipurpose catheter (MPA). A 6 mm diameter × 14 cm long Nester coil (COOK Medical) was loaded and pushed with a 0.035 in Bentson wire. There was some resistance initially but the coil was deployed satisfactorily. A second identical coil was loaded but jammed at the end of the catheter tip failing to release. The catheter had to be removed through the sheath together with the coil. To minimize the risk of losing the coil, the hub of the sheath was cut off prior to removal of the catheter and coil. On inspection the coil was seen to have exited the catheter through a side hole rather than the end hole. A side-hole catheter had been used inadvertently. Figure 1.1 shows the coil exiting through both side hole and end hole as attempts were made to push the coil out forcefully. A new sheath was placed and embolization carried out satisfactorily using an "end-hole-only" catheter.

Discussion

It is essential to use a catheter with only an end hole for the purpose of coil embolization. It is the operator's responsibility to check this prior to catheter insertion. In this case it was possible to remove the jammed coil safely along with the catheter. On occasions, coils have been lost in the venous system and had to be retrieved by snaring.

Commentary

During coil embolization procedures, coil retrieval sometimes becomes necessary for a variety of reasons.

As illustrated by the case above, end-hole-only catheters should always be used. Should a coil become trapped in a side hole, the catheter and coil should be withdrawn as suction is applied with a large syringe to minimize risk of it being "dropped" on the way back to the sheath. The coil may become lodged at the tip of the sheath in which case it can be snared close to the puncture site.

If a catheter becomes displaced with a partially deployed coil, pushing the catheter back into position may work. If not, the maneuver described above should be carried out to remove catheter and coil.

Further Reading

Huggon IC, Qureshi SA, Reidy J, et al. Percutaneous transcatheter retrieval of misplaced therapeutic embolisation devices. Br Heart J. 1994; 72(5):470–5.

Marsh P, Holdstock JM, Bacon JL, et al. Coil protruding into the common femoral vein following pelvic venous embolization. Cardiovasc Intervent Radiol. 2008;31:435–8.

Chapter 2
Retrieval of an Intravascular Foreign Body in the Venous System

Robert P. Allison, Anna Maria Belli, Joo-Young Chun, Raymond Chung, Raj Das, Andrew England, Karen Flood, Marie-France Giroux, Richard G. McWilliams, Robert Morgan, Nik Papadakos, Jai V. Patel, Raf Patel, Uday Patel, Lakshmi Ratnam, Reddi Prasad Yadavali, and John Rose

Abstract In this case, the retrieval of a "lost" guidewire from a central venous catheter placement is described. This technique is easily achievable and should be familiar to all interventional radiologists.

Keywords Complications • Foreign body retrieval • Snare

R.P. Allison
Department of Interventional Radiology,
University Hospitals Southampton,
Southampton, Hampshire, UK

A.M. Belli
Department of Radiology, St. George's Hospital
and Medical School, Blackshaw Road,
London SW17 0RE, UK
e-mail: anna.belli@stgeorges.nhs.uk

J.-Y. Chun • R. Chung
R. Das • R. Morgan • N. Papadakos
Department of Radiology, St. George's Hospital, London, UK

A. England
Department of Radiography, University of Salford,
Manchester, UK

K. Flood
Department of Vascular Radiology,
Leeds General Infirmary, Leeds, UK

M.-F. Giroux
Department of Radiology, CHUM-Centre
Hospitalier de l'Université de Montréal,
Montreal, QC, Canada

R.G. McWilliams
Department of Radiology, Royal Liverpool
University Hospital, Liverpool, UK

J.V. Patel
Department of Radiology, The Leeds Teaching
Hospitals NHS Trust, Leeds, West Yorkshire, UK

R. Patel
Department of Radiology,
The Leeds Teaching Hospitals NHS Trust ,
Leeds, West Yorkshire, UK
e-mail: rafpatel@gmail.com

U. Patel
Department of Radiology,
St. George's Hospital and Medical School,
Blackshaw Road, SW17 0QT London, UK
e-mail: uday.patel@stgeorges.nhs.uk

L. Ratnam
Department of Radiology, St. George's Hospital,
Blackshaw Road, SW17 0QT London, UK
e-mail: lakshmi.ratnam@nhs.net

R.P. Yadavali
Department of Radiology, Aberdeen Royal
Infirmary, Aberdeen, UK

J. Rose
Department of Interventional Radiology,
Freeman Hospital, Newcastle Upon Tyne
Hospitals NHS Trust, Newcastle upon Tyne, UK

Chapter 2. Retrieval of an Intravascular Foreign Body

Case History

An 80-year-old gentleman was referred to interventional radiology for retrieval of a guidewire lost into the venous system during placement of a central line. The line was placed without fluoroscopic guidance via the right internal jugular vein prior to surgery for a perforated sigmoid diverticulum.

Procedure

Fluoroscopy in the interventional suite showed the wire to have migrated inferiorly with the leading end projected over the superior aspect of the right femoral head in keeping with a location in the right common femoral vein (CFV) (Fig. 2.1a).

Ultrasound-guided access to the right CFV was performed and a 6 Fr sheath inserted.

A Multi-Snare (PFM Medical UK) with a 10–15 mm variable diameter loop was advanced through the sheath into the right CFV and distal external iliac vein to engage the leading end of the wire. The snare catheter was then advanced over the snare fixing the guidewire in position. Then maintaining traction on the snare, the snare with the engaged guidewire was retracted into the sheath and removed under fluoroscopic guidance (Fig. 2.1b). The sheath was removed and access site hemostasis achieved with manual compression.

Discussion and Tips

- It is essential to have constant control of the trailing end of a guidewire when advancing a catheter into the body.
- If a guidewire or other device is lost in the body, an interventional radiologist should be contacted in the first instance.
- There are many novel techniques reported in the literature to remove foreign bodies although snaring is the dominant strategy.
- Interventional radiologists should familiarize themselves with these techniques and the different snares available.

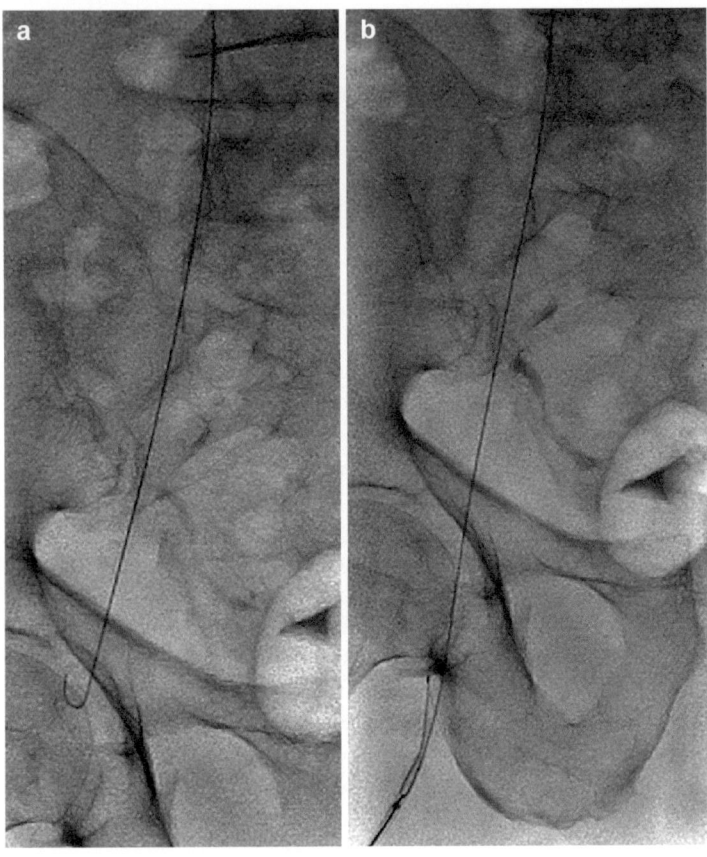

FIGURE 2.1 (**a**) Migrated wire with leading edge projected over the right common femoral head; (**b**) Snared wire being pulled into the vascular sheath

Commentary

Loop snares or goose neck snares are commonly used in retrieval of intravascular objects as they have no sharp edges and are smooth and flexible, therefore very safe. The snare loop when deployed emerges at right angles to the shaft.

Chapter 2. Retrieval of an Intravascular Foreign Body

Baskets and forceps have rigid tips and could potentially grasp the vessel wall and are therefore more hazardous to use.

Snares come in a variety of sizes. Selection of snare size is dependent on the size and location of the object being retrieved. Consideration should be given to the size of the introducer sheath being used as this should ideally accommodate the snare and the object being retrieved. As in this case, if the free end of a catheter or wire is in the IVC or inferior to that, it is relatively straightforward to snare it. The snare should be opened up below the wire and gently advanced over it. When the wire is felt to be within the snare, the loop is then tightened, and if the wire has indeed been snared, the entire assembly is withdrawn as described above. If not, the process is simply repeated until the wire is snared, varying the position of the snare by rotation at the hub.

When there is no free edge to be grasped, the foreign body can be displaced or moved to where there is adequate space for the snare loop to form. One of the commonest foreign body retrievals is catheter fragments in the heart. These can be pulled down into the IVC using a pigtail catheter. A pigtail catheter is advanced close to the fragment and looped over it either by rotating the pigtail or using the guidewire to get the pigtail to form over the foreign body. It is then pulled down into the IVC where a snare can be used to grasp the free edge.

For objects with a hollow center and vertical orientation (e.g., a stent), a "coaxial" snare technique can be employed. The snare loop is placed over a guidewire and then these are introduced together into the vascular sheath. The guidewire is then passed through the middle of the tubular object being snared. The snare loop is then "walked" over the guidewire to surround the object being snared before the loop is then tightened around the foreign body. This has the advantage of improved alignment of the snared object with the sheath thus facilitating retrieval.

The snare technique is relatively easy to master with a high rate of success and low complication rates.

Further Reading

Carroll MI, Ahanchi SS, Kim JH, et al. Endovascular foreign body retrieval. J Vasc Surg. 2013;57(2):459–63.

Schechter MA, O'Brien PJ, Cox MW. Retrieval of iatrogenic intravascular foreign bodies. J Vasc Surg. 2013;57(1):276–81.

Woodhouse JB, Uberoi R. Techniques for intravascular foreign body retrieval. Cardiovasc Intervent Radiol. 2013;36(4):888–97.

Chapter 3
Migrated Superior Vena Cava Stent Repositioned Using a Balloon and Loop Snare Combination

Robert P. Allison, Anna Maria Belli, Joo-Young Chun, Raymond Chung, Raj Das, Andrew England, Karen Flood, Marie-France Giroux, Richard G. McWilliams, Robert Morgan, Nik Papadakos, Jai V. Patel, Raf Patel, Uday Patel, Lakshmi Ratnam, Reddi Prasad Yadavali, and John Rose

Abstract This case describes the snaring and repositioning of a migrated SVC stent. Various other techniques for managing this complication are also discussed.

Keywords Complication • SVC stent migration • Snare

R.P. Allison
Department of Interventional Radiology, University Hospitals Southampton, Southampton, Hampshire, UK

A.M. Belli
Department of Radiology, St. George's Hospital and Medical School, Blackshaw Road, London SW17 0RE, UK
e-mail: anna.belli@stgeorges.nhs.uk

J.-Y. Chun • R. Chung
R. Das • R. Morgan • N. Papadakos
Department of Radiology, St. George's Hospital, London, UK

L. Ratnam et al. (eds.), *Managing Common Interventional Radiology Complications*, DOI 10.1007/978-1-4471-5502-7_3,
© Springer-Verlag London 2014

A. England
Department of Radiography, University
of Salford, Manchester, UK

K. Flood
Department of Vascular Radiology,
Leeds General Infirmary, Leeds, UK

M.-F. Giroux
Department of Radiology, CHUM-Centre
Hospitalier de l'Université de Montréal,
Montreal, QC, Canada

R.G. McWilliams
Department of Radiology, Royal Liverpool
University Hospital, Liverpool, UK

J.V. Patel
Department of Radiology, The Leeds Teaching
Hospitals NHS Trust, Leeds, West Yorkshire, UK

R. Patel
Department of Radiology,
The Leeds Teaching Hospitals NHS Trust,
Leeds, West Yorkshire, UK
e-mail: rafpatel@gmail.com

U. Patel
Department of Diagnostic Radiology,
St. George's Hospital and Medical School,
Blackshaw Road, SW17 0QT London, UK
e-mail: uday.patel@stgeorges.nhs.uk

L. Ratnam
Department of Radiology, St. George's Hospital,
Blackshaw Road, SW17 0QT London, UK
e-mail: lakshmi.ratnam@nhs.net

R.P. Yadavali
Department of Radiology, Aberdeen Royal
Infirmary, Aberdeen, UK

J. Rose
Department of Interventional Radiology,
Freeman Hospital, Newcastle Upon Tyne
Hospitals NHS Trust, Newcastle upon Tyne, UK

Case History

A 33-year-old man was referred for bilateral upper limb and central venography to identify potential new sites for arteriovenous fistulae (AVF). He had chronic renal failure secondary to reflux nephropathy and a complex surgical history including failed cadaveric renal transplant and multiple failed limb AVFs.

Venography demonstrated poor peripheral veins, occlusion of the left subclavian vein, and a distal SVC stenosis with large azygos vein. The patient proceeded to SVC stent insertion to facilitate the success of a planned right arm AVF.

Procedure

Using a micropuncture kit, the right subclavian vein (SCV) was cannulated laterally under ultrasound guidance. The distal SVC stenosis was pre-dilated with an 8-mm balloon which clearly showed a short focal tight stenosis of approximately 1 cm in length (Fig. 3.1a, b). A 16×60-mm WALLSTENT (Boston Scientific, Galway, Ireland) was inserted and post-dilated to 12 mm (Fig. 3.2a).

As ongoing dialysis was required and both internal jugular veins and the left subclavian vein were occluded, a central line insertion was attempted from the right subclavian vein. This proved to be a difficult procedure as the central line would not track easily over the guidewire and advancing the dual lumen central line resulted in dislodgement of the Wallstent and subsequent migration into the right atrium (Fig. 3.2b).

At this stage, right common femoral vein access was obtained and a 14-Fr sheath inserted. Through-and-through wire access to secure the stent was obtained by passing a guidewire from the right SCV through the stent, snaring it in the IVC and pulling it out through the femoral sheath.

A 25-mm Amplatz GooseNeck snare (Bard, USA) was preloaded onto an 18-mm balloon which was then passed into the stent over the guidewire (Fig. 3.3a). The balloon was partially inflated in the stent, and the Gooseneck snare then easily slid over the balloon and onto the stent from below (Fig. 3.3b).

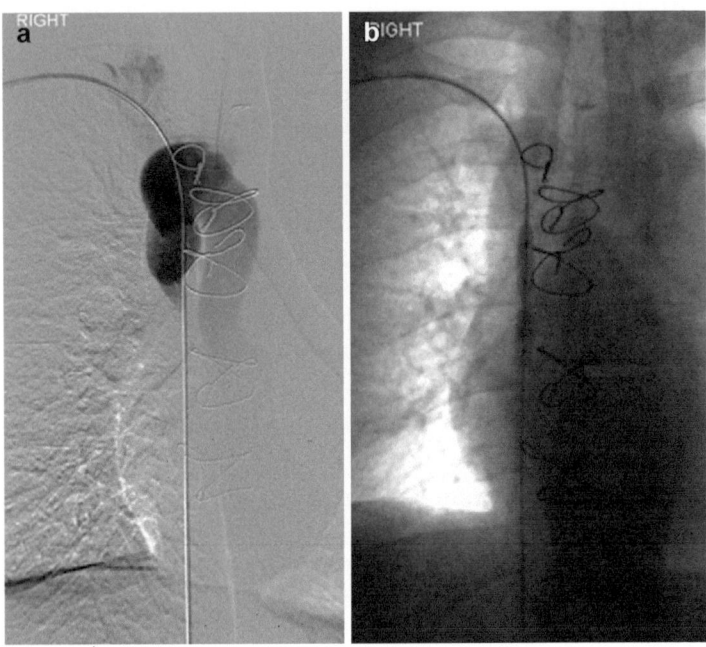

FIGURE 3.1 (**a**) Distal SVC stenosis; (**b**) stenosis length defined by balloon dilatation

The entire assembly of stent, snare, and balloon was then pulled down into the right common iliac vein (Fig. 3.3c). Venoplasty of the stent in the right iliac vein was performed to 12 mm to secure it in place. A right femoral Vas Cath was inserted into the right common femoral vein, through the stent and the tip placed in the IVC for dialysis requirements until the AVF was formed.

Discussion

Stenting of the superior vena cava (SVC) is an accepted treatment for SVC obstruction and is mostly performed for malignant obstruction. Symptoms of SVC obstruction include dyspnea, dysphagia, headaches, and reduced cognitive function with clinical signs of arm, neck, and facial swelling, plethora,

Chapter 3. Migrated Superior Vena Cava Stent 17

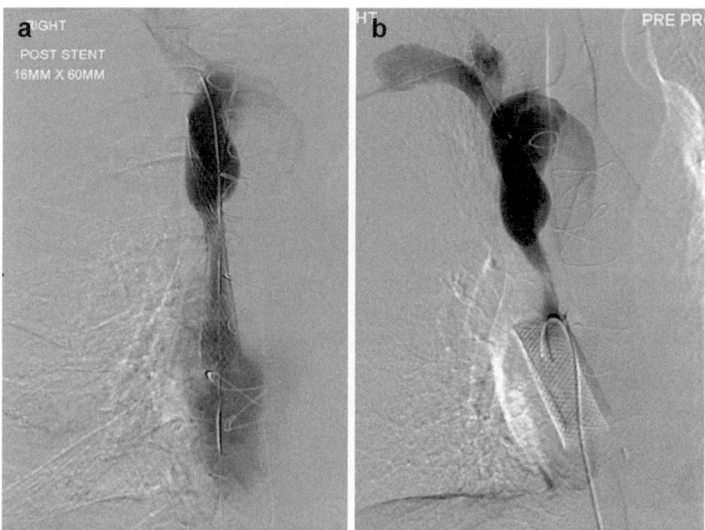

FIGURE 3.2 (**a**) Stent position post-deployment; (**b**) displaced stent in the right atrium

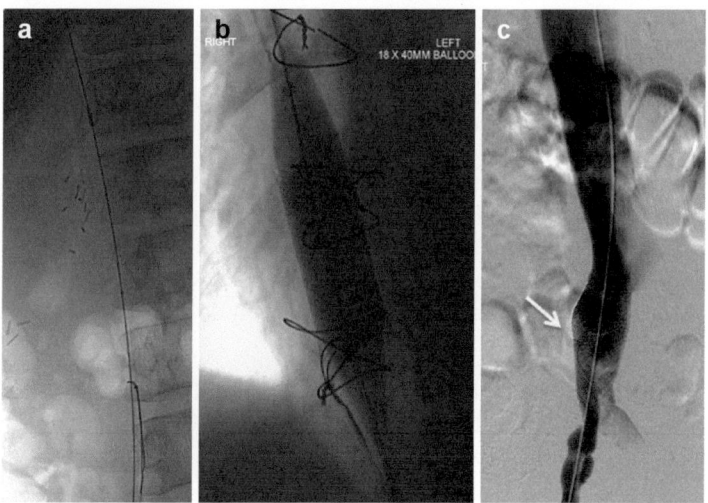

FIGURE 3.3 (**a**) Snare placed over balloon catheter external to the patient then advanced as a single unit over the wire; (**b**) with the balloon partially inflated, the snare catheter easily slides over the tapered end of the balloon and over the stent; (**c**) final position of the stent in the right common iliac vein (*arrow*)

and distended veins in the chest wall and neck. Emergency intervention is considered in cases of reduced consciousness or dyspnea. Indications for SVC stenting have now extended to include benign disorders such as central venous strictures from hemodialysis catheters. Caution is advised in treatment of malignancy with good chance of cure or remission and in benign disease where there is a long life expectancy.

The overall complication rate of 5.8–7 % includes restenosis and thrombosis, SVC rupture, pericardial tamponade, pulmonary emboli/infarction, stent migration, cardiac failure, respiratory failure, acute pulmonary edema, hemorrhage, hemoptysis, epistaxis, recurrent laryngeal palsy, and infection. Stent migration is reported in approximately 2 % of case and renders the patient susceptible to potentially life-threatening complications unless the stent is retrieved and repositioned or stabilized.

Techniques designed to minimize the risk of migration include deploying the majority of the stent on the peripheral side of the lesion, avoiding stent placement around sharp curves, adequate stent oversizing to increase the expansile force of the stent against vessel wall, and retaining a slight "waist" in the center to prevent stent migration by allowing the flared ends to become slightly embedded in the vein wall.

Retrieval technique depends on the final stent positioning and the ability to snare the stent.

The stent is first secured by passing a guidewire through the stent lumen and exiting through two separate venous access points, commonly the right internal jugular and common femoral vein vascular sheaths. This helps prevent further movement into the right cardiac chambers and pulmonary arterial outflow tract. Once this has been done, there are several possibilities.

- Using an angioplasty balloon to assist in snaring the stent as described in the case above.
- Utilizing multiple overlapping stents to stabilize the migrated stent resulting in a SVC to IVC stent "bridge."
- Directly snaring the stent over the stabilizing guidewire with a 25-mm Amplatz Gooseneck snare (Bard, USA) and repositioning the stent in the common iliac vein.

- If it proves impossible to lasso the stent with the snare, grasping the end of the stent with an intravascular biopsy forceps and repositioning it in a larger caliber vessel have been described.

In the event of difficult withdrawal of the stent through the vascular sheath, following successful snaring, options include deployment in a safe venous location such as the iliac vein, elongating the stent with a second snare by pulling from both ends via two access points before removing it through one of the vascular sheaths, or removal via a surgical venotomy.

Tips

- Stent length should include at least 10 mm free at either end of the obstruction.
- Dilatation of the stent post-deployment assists early full stent expansion rather than relying on the stent's inherent radial force alone.
- Combined radiological and surgical approaches may be necessary to ensure safe retrieval while maintaining important venous access in a complex patient cohort likely facing multiple future vascular access procedures.

Commentary

SVC stenting is usually a straightforward procedure, but stent migration is a well recognized complication experienced by many IRs during their practice. It is essential to stabilize the stent and keep the guidewire through the stent to avoid it tilting in the right atrium. Ideally it should be repositioned, but "bridge" stenting from the SVC to IVC is easy to perform if the wire remains in place. Sometimes fixing the stent with another stent in the brachiocephalic vein is required if the stent position does not seem stable and this will prevent late migration.

Further Reading

Taylor JD, Lehmann ED, Belli A-M, Nicholson AA, Kessel D, Robertson IR, Pollock JG, Morgan RA. Strategies for the management of SVC stent migration into the right atrium. Cardiovasc Intervent Radiol. 2007;30:1003–9.

Uberoi R. Quality assurance guidelines for superior vena cava stenting in malignant disease. Cardiovasc Intervent Radiol. 2006;29:319–22.

Chapter 4
Retrieval of Central Venous Catheter Fragment Following Portacath Removal

Robert P. Allison, Anna Maria Belli, Joo-Young Chun, Raymond Chung, Raj Das, Andrew England, Karen Flood, Marie-France Giroux, Richard G. McWilliams, Robert Morgan, Nik Papadakos, Jai V. Patel, Raf Patel, Uday Patel, Lakshmi Ratnam, Reddi Prasad Yadavali, and John Rose

Abstract This case describes retrieval of a retained segment of central line from an implanted port device. The variation in technique required for retrieval which may be influenced by the material of the retained fragment is also discussed.

Keywords Complication • Foreign body retrieval • Snare • Central venous catheter

---

R.P. Allison
Department of Interventional Radiology,
University Hospitals Southampton,
Southampton, Hampshire, UK

A.M. Belli
Department of Radiology, St. George's
Hospital and Medical School, Blackshaw
Road, London SW17 0RE, UK
e-mail: anna.belli@stgeorges.nhs.uk

J.-Y. Chun • R. Chung
R. Das • R. Morgan • N. Papadakos
Department of Radiology, St. George's Hospital, London, UK

A. England
Department of Radiography, University of Salford, Manchester, UK

K. Flood
Department of Vascular Radiology,
Leeds General Infirmary, Leeds, UK

M.-F. Giroux
Department of Radiology, CHUM-Centre
Hospitalier de l'Université de Montréal,
Montreal, QC, Canada

R.G. McWilliams
Department of Radiology, Royal Liverpool
University Hospital, Liverpool, UK

J.V. Patel
Department of Radiology, The Leeds Teaching
Hospitals NHS Trust, Leeds, West Yorkshire, UK

R. Patel
Department of Radiology,
The Leeds Teaching Hospitals NHS Trust,
Leeds, West Yorkshire, UK
e-mail: rafpatel@gmail.com

U. Patel
Department of Diagnostic Radiology,
St. George's Hospital and Medical School,
Blackshaw Road, SW17 0QT London, UK
e-mail: uday.patel@stgeorges.nhs.uk

L. Ratnam
Department of Radiology, St. George's Hospital,
Blackshaw Road, SW17 0QT London, UK
e-mail: lakshmi.ratnam@nhs.net

R.P. Yadavali
Department of Radiology, Aberdeen Royal
Infirmary, Aberdeen, UK

J. Rose
Department of Interventional Radiology,
Freeman Hospital, Newcastle Upon Tyne
Hospitals NHS Trust, Newcastle upon Tyne, UK

Case History

A 67-year-old female with chronic kidney disease and a history of multiple failed arteriovenous (AV) fistulae had no further potential options for AV fistula formation. A Dialock port was placed in the right subclavian vein to allow access for hemodialysis. Six weeks following placement of the port, there was malfunction of the port and it was surgically removed. However, only one of the port lumens could be retrieved. A chest X-ray demonstrated the remaining lumen had detached and lay within the right central venous system. Following discussion of possible management options, endovascular retrieval of the retained lumen offered the least invasive option.

Procedure

A 12F sheath was placed in the right internal jugular vein, and venography demonstrated the proximal end of the port lumen embedded in the wall of the right brachiocephalic vein (Fig. 4.1a). The distal end lay free in the right atrium (RA). To free up the proximal end, a gooseneck snare was passed around the distal end in the right atrium and the port lumen "pushed" further into the RA. The snare was loosened and repositioned over the proximal tip of the port lumen in order to pull the lumen through the access sheath. However, due to slight tilting of the port lumen by the snare, there was malalignment of the port lumen with respect to the sheath lumen, and so retrieval was not possible. A Berenstein catheter and Terumo wire were then used to pass a guidewire into the port lumen (Fig. 4.1b). This was exchanged for a low profile 2 mm × 10 cm angioplasty balloon which was placed partially into the port lumen and inflated (Fig. 4.2a). The gooseneck snare was then coaxially passed over the balloon catheter, in order to snare the proximal end of the port (Fig. 4.2b). The port was then pulled up to the sheath, using the angioplasty balloon to align the proximal tip of the port lumen with the tip of the sheath lumen and "guide" it into the sheath to enable its removal.

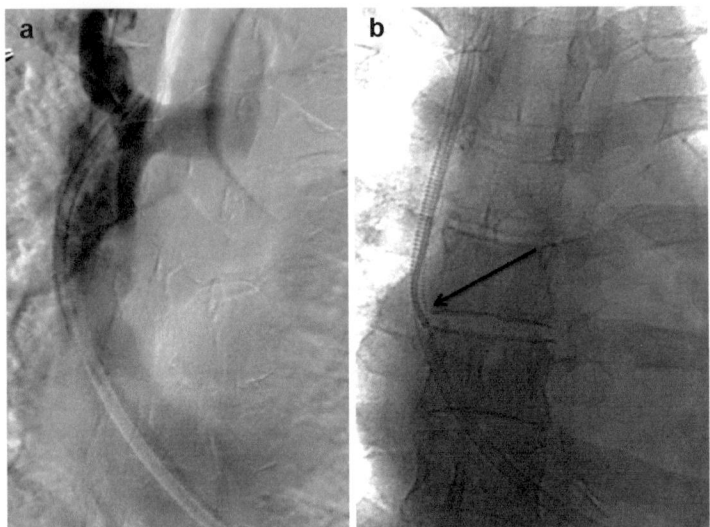

FIGURE 4.1 (**a**) Detached Dialock catheter. Venogram demonstrated the proximal end embedded in the wall of the right brachiocephalic vein and the distal end free in the right atrium; (**b**) a Berenstein catheter (*arrow*) has been passed down the center of the port lumen

Once the fragment had been removed, a tunnelled Tesio line was placed as an alternative access for hemodialysis.

Discussion

Tunnelled central venous access lines are frequently used in the hemodialysis population when options for an arteriovenous fistula have been exhausted. Infection of lines remains a major drawback to their use. In an attempt to reduce infection rates, implantable ports have been utilized for long-term hemodialysis access. The Dialock is one such device which consists of a subcutaneous chamber attached to two reinforced port lumens. The port lumens are fairly inflexible and, thus, require insertion via a subclavian vein approach. In addition to the standard complications of tunnelled central venous catheters, such as line blockage from

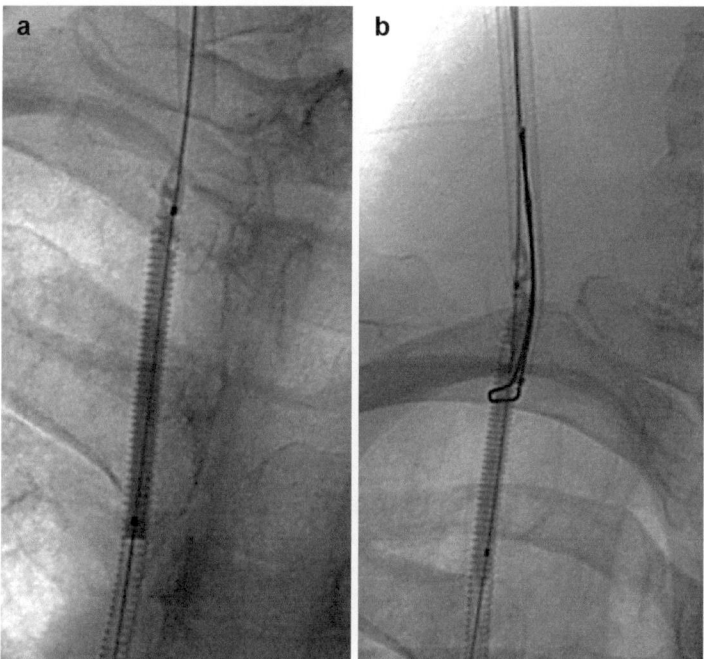

FIGURE 4.2 (**a**) A low profile balloon was placed partially into the port lumen and inflated. This allowed the proximal end of the lumen to remain aligned to the venous sheath during removal of the port lumen; (**b**) a gooseneck snare was placed over the port lumen. The whole assembly was pulled into the venous sheath and the port lumen retrieved

fibrin sheath and pericatheter thrombus formation, with implantable ports, there is the potential for the port lumen to detach from the chamber.

Venous access ports are utilized in a number of patient groups. The majority of these devices have very flexible port lumens which allow retrieval of detached lumen by standard snaring techniques. Those ports with more rigid lumen, such as the Dialock, require modification of technique to allow their successful removal by endovascular techniques. This case demonstrates one such modification used to retrieve a port lumen which detached during attempted surgical removal.

Tips

- Foreign bodies from fragments of venous catheters and ports and guidewires should not be left in situ as they can migrate into the pulmonary arteries and perforate the heart or vessels.
- Knowledge of the type of catheter/port is important as fragments from standard ports which are flexible, e.g., portacath, can be retrieved by snaring one free end as the segment is flexible enough to loop as it is withdrawn and removed through an oversized access sheath.
- Ports with a reinforced lumen, e.g., Dialock, do not readily bend and require modifications in technique to align the proximal end of the port lumen with the access sheath lumen during retrieval.
- Angioplasty balloons, with their "shouldered" ends are ideal for allowing a smoother transition between a rigid port lumen and the sheath, aiding their removal.
- Cutting the tip of the sheath obliquely may facilitate withdrawal of such catheters into the sheath.

Commentary

Foreign body retrieval from the venous or arterial system is a fundamental skill for interventional radiologists as the alternative surgical techniques are much more invasive.

Foreign bodies in the venous system can migrate into the pulmonary arteries and should be retrieved as they can cause infection, myocardial or valvular perforation, arrhythmias, and death.

There are a variety of methods described for removal. Soft catheters with a free end can be snared and withdrawn into a larger sheath. Entry into the sheath can be improved by cutting the aperture obliquely before insertion. When the foreign body is rigid, this may still not pass into the sheath easily, and the method described here allows alignment and retrieval. The combined and coaxial use of a balloon catheter and loop snare can also be used to aid snaring of wayward stents, as described in the previous case, and other hollow fragments.

Further Reading

Cahill AM, Ballah D, Hernandez P, Fontalvo L. Percutaneous retrieval of intravascular venous foreign bodies in children. Pediatr Radiol. 2012;42(1):24–31. doi:10.1007/s00247-011-2150-z. Epub 2011 Dec 17.

Cheng CC, Tsai TN, Yang CC, Han CL. Percutaneous retrieval of dislodged totally implantable central venous access system in 92 cases: experience in a single hospital. Eur J Radiol. 2009;69(2):346–50.

Surov A, Wienke A, Carter JM, Stoevesandt D, Behrmann C, Spielmann RP, Werdan K, Buerke M. Intravascular embolization of venous catheter–causes, clinical signs, and management: a systematic review. J Parenter Enteral Nutr. 2009;33(6):677–85.

Chapter 5
Central Venous Catheter Inserted into the Mediastinum

Robert P. Allison, Anna Maria Belli, Joo-Young Chun, Raymond Chung, Raj Das, Andrew England, Karen Flood, Marie-France Giroux, Richard G. McWilliams, Robert Morgan, Nik Papadakos, Jai V. Patel, Raf Patel, Uday Patel, Lakshmi Ratnam, Reddi Prasad Yadavali, and John Rose

Abstract This case discusses the management of a misplaced central venous line including the diagnostic difficulties this may present in determining the exact location of a line which is not in its intended location.

Keywords Central venous line • Complications • Mediastinal rupture • Misplaced

R.P. Allison
Department of Interventional Radiology,
University Hospitals Southampton,
Southampton, Hampshire, UK

A.M. Belli
Department of Radiology, St. George's
Hospital and Medical School, Blackshaw
Road, London SW17 0RE, UK
e-mail: anna.belli@stgeorges.nhs.uk

L. Ratnam et al. (eds.), *Managing Common Interventional Radiology Complications*, DOI 10.1007/978-1-4471-5502-7_5,
© Springer-Verlag London 2014

J.-Y. Chun • R. Chung
R. Das • R. Morgan • N. Papadakos
Department of Radiology, St. George's Hospital, London, UK

A. England
Department of Radiography, University of Salford, Manchester, UK

K. Flood
Department of Vascular Radiology,
Leeds General Infirmary, Leeds, UK

M.-F. Giroux
Department of Radiology, CHUM-Centre
Hospitalier de l'Université de Montréal,
Montreal, QC, Canada

R.G. McWilliams
Department of Radiology, Royal Liverpool
University Hospital, Liverpool, UK

J.V. Patel
Department of Radiology, The Leeds Teaching
Hospitals NHS Trust, Leeds, West Yorkshire, UK

R. Patel
Department of Radiology,
The Leeds Teaching Hospitals NHS Trust,
Leeds, West Yorkshire, UK
e-mail: rafpatel@gmail.com

U. Patel
Department of Diagnostic Radiology,
St. George's Hospital and Medical School,
Blackshaw Road, SW17 0QT London, UK
e-mail: uday.patel@stgeorges.nhs.uk

L. Ratnam
Department of Radiology, St. George's Hospital,
Blackshaw Road, SW17 0QT London, UK
e-mail: lakshmi.ratnam@nhs.net

R.P. Yadavali
Department of Radiology, Aberdeen Royal
Infirmary, Aberdeen, UK

J. Rose
Department of Interventional Radiology,
Freeman Hospital, Newcastle Upon Tyne
Hospitals NHS Trust, Newcastle upon Tyne, UK

Chapter 5. Misplaced Central Venous Catheter

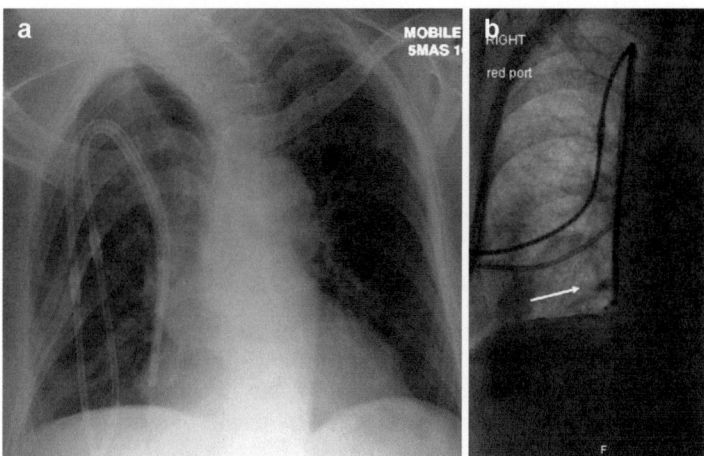

FIGURE 5.1 (**a**) CXR showing very lateral position of CVC; (**b**) linogram showing contrast extravasation into the thoracic cavity (*arrow*)

Case History

A 48-year-old woman underwent an ultrasound-guided insertion of a right internal jugular dual lumen Tesio® (Medcomp, Harleysville, PA, USA) central venous catheter (CVC) for hemodialysis. Following cannulation, blood could not be withdrawn from the line. Routine CXR showed lateral positioning of the CVC (Fig. 5.1a) and a linogram was arranged.

Procedure

Contrast injected via the line was seen to extravasate into the right hemithorax via both lumens (Fig. 5.1b). An urgent CT scan of the thorax was performed which confirmed the catheter was outside the vascular space, though the exact site of perforation could not be identified (Fig. 5.2a).

Arteriography (Fig. 5.2b) did not reveal arterial injury. On venography (Fig. 5.2c), the site of perforation could not be confidently identified, though it was suspected to be from the right brachiocephalic vein.

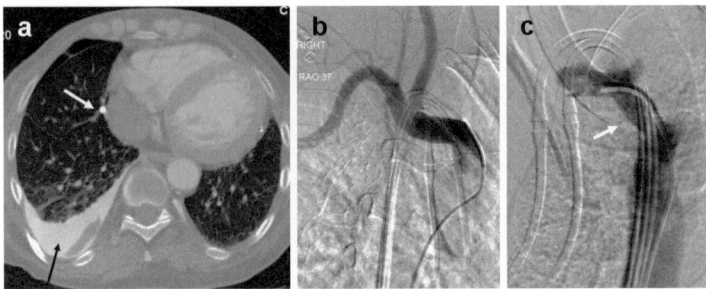

Figure 5.2 (**a**) CT of the thorax showing the tip of the CVC lying outside the vena cava with the tip in lower medial pleural space (*white arrow*). There is associated contrast and hematoma in the pleural space (*black arrow*), with a small pneumothorax; (**b**) Initial arteriography revealed no injury; (**c**) Initial venography did not show definite site of perforation but suspected contrast extravasation from the brachiocephalic vein as shown (*arrow*)

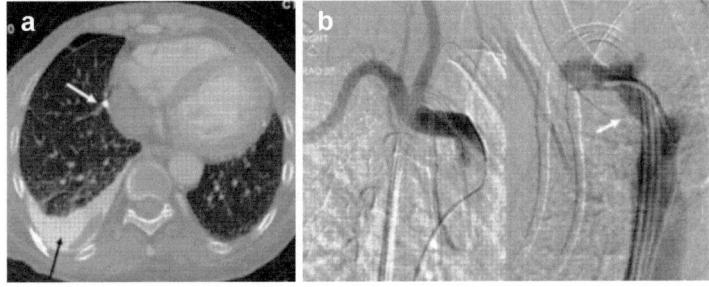

Figure 5.3 (**a**) Post-stenting imaging of the right brachiocephalic vein with no extravasation of contrast; (**b**) C-arm CT confirming increasing hemothorax despite stenting, and an ultrasound-guided chest drain was immediately inserted

After discussion with the cardiothoracic surgical team, an Atrium Advanta™ V12 balloon expandable covered stent (Atrium Medical Corporation, Hudson, NH, USA) was deployed in the right brachiocephalic vein (Fig. 5.3a). The stent was positioned to avoid covering the contralateral brachiocephalic vein and appeared adequately placed with no evidence of hemorrhage, but as soon as the venous catheter was removed, the right hemithorax was seen to fill with blood during screening and confirmed on C-arm CT (Fig. 5.3b). A US-guided chest drain was inserted and the cardiothoracic surgeons were contacted. An emergency posterolateral thoracotomy was performed, and the perforation was identified at the junction of the brachiocephalic vein and SVC, which was repaired. The patient was discharged 6 weeks postoperatively with no long-term complications.

Discussion

Hemothorax is a known serious complication of CVC insertion and thought to be a more significantly prognostic indicator of death than any other CVC complication combined. Hemothorax secondary to arterial injury is the most commonly reported cause, with a number of case reports describing successful endovascular stenting.

Venous injury resulting in hemothorax is rare. The sites of injury described include the SVC, subclavian, and brachiocephalic veins. These are caused by direct injury to the vessel wall by the guidewire or dilator. Due to vasospasm in the vein wall and its lower venous pressures, venous injury is less likely to manifest with a rapid or significant amount of blood loss, as in arterial injury. This, along with underreporting, may mean that such injuries are rarely detected; hence, the true incidence is unknown. Arterial injury is far more common and well described in the literature. The successful use of covered stents and vascular closure devices to manage arterial perforation has also been reported.

Successful endovascular stenting of an SVC perforation following CVC insertion has been previously reported. Our attempt at stenting was unsuccessful as the perforation, being at the junction of the brachiocephalic vein and SVC, was not recognized at the time and the position of the stent did not cover the site of perforation. In addition the caliber difference of the vessels that the stent was placed across may also have resulted in suboptimal stent conformity.

In retrospect a number of alterative techniques could have been employed; for example, we could have withdrawn the CVC line with simultaneous contrast injection in an attempt to identify the exact site of perforation and allow for a subsequent more accurate stent placement. Also the CVC could have been withdrawn after the initial stent was placed and a further stent introduced if the hemorrhage had continued or the stent was shown not to have achieved optimal coverage. Alternatively if the site of perforation had not been clearly identified, then additional proximal stenting in an attempt to achieve maximal coverage could have been considered although there would be a risk of covering the contralateral vein.

We have subsequently established protocols to manage this serious CVC-related complication and suggest close liaison between the interventional radiologists and cardiothoracic surgeons.

Tips

- Appreciate that large and central vein perforation secondary to CVC misplacement can carry significant morbidity and mortality.
- The line should not be removed and early diagnosis with a linogram and CT should be arranged.
- Early liaison with the cardiothoracic team should be sought in the event of an IR procedure failing to stop the hemorrhage.
- The line should only be removed when the exact site of perforation is identified prior to or during stent insertion.
- Be prepared to use more than one covered stent if the hemorrhage continues.

Commentary

This case highlights an increasingly recognized complication of central line placement. The venogram after placement of the covered stent shows that the stent probably did not extend far enough, as the perforation was at the junction with the SVC. This is potentially a difficult site to seal a perforation because of the large change in caliber of the veins. However, contrast injection through the catheter as it was being removed would have helped confirm the exact site of perforation. Even if a second stent-graft had been placed unsuccessfully, an occlusion balloon could have tamponaded the site of bleeding and reduced hemorrhage into the thorax while awaiting surgery. Arterial closure devices have been used successfully in arteries but not in veins.

Further Reading

Azizzadeh A, Pham MT, Estrera AL, Coogan SM, Safi HJ. Endovascular repair of an iatrogenic superior vena caval injury: a case report. J Vasc Surg. 2007;46(3):569–71.

Domino KB, Bowdle TA, Posner KL, Spitellie PH, Lee LA, Cheney FW. Injuries and liability related to central vascular catheters: a closed claims analysis. Anesthesiology. 2004;100(6):1411–8.

Guilbert MC, Elkouri S, Bracco D, Corriveau MM, Beaudoin N, Dubois MJ, Bruneau L, Blair JF. Arterial trauma during central venous catheter insertion: case series, review and proposed algorithm. J Vasc Surg. 2008;48(4):918–25.

Shetty SV, Kwolek CJ, Garasic JM. Percutaneous closure after inadvertent subclavian artery cannulation. Catheter Cardiovasc Interv. 2007; 69(7):1050–2.

Chapter 6
Femoral Artery Pseudoaneurysm Treated with Percutaneous Thrombin Injection

Robert P. Allison, Anna Maria Belli, Joo-Young Chun, Raymond Chung, Raj Das, Andrew England, Karen Flood, Marie-France Giroux, Richard G. McWilliams, Robert Morgan, Nik Papadakos, Jai V. Patel, Raf Patel, Uday Patel, Lakshmi Ratnam, Reddi Prasad Yadavali, and John Rose

Abstract This case illustrates the treatment of a post-femoral artery catheterization pseudoaneurysm with ultrasound-guided thrombin injection. Images illustrate the diagnosis and posttreatment appearances.

Keywords Angiography • Complications • Pseudoaneurysm • Thrombin

---

R.P. Allison
Department of Interventional Radiology, University Hospitals Southampton, Southampton, Hampshire, UK

A.M. Belli
Department of Radiology, St. George's Hospital and Medical School, Blackshaw Road, London SW17 0RE, UK
e-mail: anna.belli@stgeorges.nhs.uk

J.-Y. Chun • R. Chung
R. Das • R. Morgan • N. Papadakos
Department of Radiology, St. George's Hospital, London, UK
A. England
Department of Radiography, University of Salford, Manchester, UK

K. Flood
Department of Vascular Radiology,
Leeds General Infirmary, Leeds, UK

M.-F. Giroux
Department of Radiology, CHUM-Centre
Hospitalier de l'Université de Montréal,
Montreal, QC, Canada

R.G. McWilliams
Department of Radiology, Royal Liverpool
University Hospital, Liverpool, UK

J.V. Patel
Department of Radiology, The Leeds Teaching
Hospitals NHS Trust, Leeds, West Yorkshire, UK

R. Patel
Department of Radiology,
The Leeds Teaching Hospitals NHS Trust,
Leeds, West Yorkshire, UK
e-mail: rafpatel@gmail.com

U. Patel
Department of Diagnostic Radiology,
St. George's Hospital and Medical School,
Blackshaw Road, SW17 0QT London, UK
e-mail: uday.patel@stgeorges.nhs.uk

L. Ratnam
Department of Radiology, St. George's Hospital,
Blackshaw Road, SW17 0QT London, UK
e-mail: lakshmi.ratnam@nhs.net

R.P. Yadavali
Department of Radiology, Aberdeen Royal
Infirmary, Aberdeen, UK

J. Rose
Department of Interventional Radiology,
Freeman Hospital, Newcastle Upon Tyne
Hospitals NHS Trust, Newcastle upon Tyne, UK

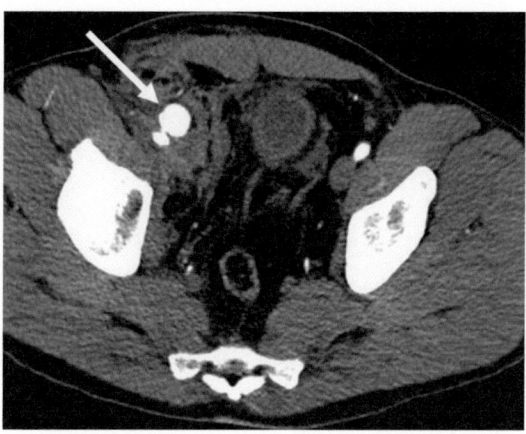

FIGURE 6.1 Axial contrast-enhanced CT demonstrates a pseudoaneurysm (*arrow*) arising from the right external iliac/common femoral artery junction

Case History

A 74-year-old male presented with chest pain and shortness of breath. ECG confirmed acute ST-elevation myocardial infarction. Emergency cardiac catheterization was performed via a right femoral approach. A significant stenosis of the left anterior descending artery was treated with angioplasty and stent deployment. No immediate complications were apparent.

Day 3 post-procedure on the coronary care unit, extensive bruising was visible in the right femoral region, and it was noted that the patient's hemoglobin had dropped from 11.4 g/dl pre-procedure to 8.7 g/dl on day 3. A puncture site complication such as a retroperitoneal hematoma or a pseudoaneurysm was suspected clinically, and an urgent CT with contrast was performed (Fig. 6.1). CT confirmed a 3.4 × 2.8 cm pseudoaneurysm arising from the junction of the right external iliac artery and the common femoral artery. Urgent ultrasound-guided thrombin injection of the pseudoaneurysm was arranged.

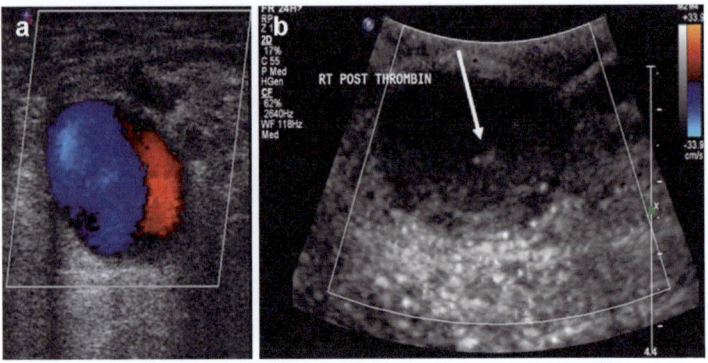

FIGURE 6.2 (**a**) Color Doppler ultrasound demonstrates characteristic bidirectional flow in the pseudoaneurysm sac; (**b**) color Doppler ultrasound demonstrates the tip of the needle (*arrow*) located in the pseudoaneurysm sac and total absence of flow in the pseudoaneurysm sac immediately after thrombin injection

Procedure

Color Doppler ultrasound confirmed characteristic bidirectional flow within an echolucent cavity communicating with the underlying artery, in keeping with a pseudoaneurysm (Fig. 6.2a). The peripheral pulses were examined and documented. A pulse oximeter probe was also placed on the right hallux prior to the procedure. Under sterile conditions and continuous ultrasound guidance, a 20 G needle was inserted into the pseudoaneurysm sac, and 400 IU of human thrombin (0.4 ml of 1,000 IU/ml) was injected slowly with constant color Doppler ultrasound monitoring. The injection was terminated when thrombosis of the pseudoaneurysm was demonstrated (Fig. 6.2b). Continuous pulse oximetry of the hallux was unchanged, and peripheral pulses and perfusion were also reexamined to exclude distal embolization. The patient was observed on bed rest on the ward post-procedure, and a follow-up ultrasound was organized for the following day. Repeat ultrasound confirmed complete thrombosis of the pseudoaneurysm with preserved patency of the underlying artery.

Discussion

Iatrogenic pseudoaneurysms occur due to inadequate hemostasis at the arterial puncture site. Extravasation of blood from the puncture site forms a pulsatile cavity in the perivascular soft tissues surrounded by hematoma and fascial layers, but not contained by any layers of the vessel wall. The main preventable risk factors for pseudoaneurysm formation are poor puncture and compression techniques. Pseudoaneurysms occur more frequently following a low superficial or profunda femoris puncture when the artery cannot be compressed against the femoral head. A high puncture above the inguinal ligament may also result in a pseudoaneurysm as illustrated above, and the danger is a much larger retroperitoneal hematoma may accumulate in the pelvic cavity before any complication is detected. Other risk factors for pseudoaneurysm formation are the use of anticoagulants and thrombolytics, larger sheath sizes (>7 Fr), obesity, and hypertension.

Femoral pseudoaneurysms are suspected clinically following arterial punctures when there is a pulsatile groin mass, and they can be easily confirmed with Doppler ultrasound.

Treatment options are conservative, ultrasound-guided compression, ultrasound-guided thrombin injection, and surgery. Conservative treatment with interval ultrasound follow-up in 7–10 days is considered for small pseudoaneurysms (less than 2 cm sac size) with no other adverse features such as skin compromise, compression of adjacent neurovascular structures, distal embolization, persistent pain, or infection. Ultrasound can be used to guide compression of the neck of the pseudoaneurysm to prevent flow in the pseudoaneurysm sac leading to thrombosis. However, this technique has a high technical failure and recurrence rate, especially in anticoagulated patients, and it is also prolonged and painful (both for the patient and the operator).

Ultrasound-guided thrombin injection is a quick, pain-free, reliable, and safe way of treating pseudoaneurysms even when patients are anticoagulated. This is now the preferred treatment modality for the majority of femoral pseudoaneurysms.

Complications related to human thrombin injection (e.g., available as Tisseel™, Baxter, Glendale, CA – unlicensed use) are reported to be rare but can include parent vessel thrombosis and distal embolization. To prevent this, very small aliquots of thrombin (0.1 ml) are injected slowly into the sac until thrombosis of the pseudoaneurysm and adjacent neck is seen on color Doppler ultrasound. Pseudoaneurysms with relatively narrow and long necks are preferred although those with short and wider necks can be treated sometimes with the addition of occlusive balloon inflation in the parent artery during thrombin injection. There is a risk of severe anaphylaxis with thrombin, more likely with bovine thrombin in patients who have previously been exposed to it rather than with recombinant human thrombin. Also rare, but a potentially significant complication, is the formation of antibodies following repeated exposure to bovine thrombin that may cross-react with human thrombin and factor V resulting in abnormalities of hemostasis.

Surgical treatment for femoral pseudoaneurysms is usually reserved for when repeated minimally invasive options have failed or there is another indication for surgery such as skin compromise, neurovascular compression, or infection when percutaneous treatment is contraindicated.

Tips

- Meticulous care and attention to detail during arterial puncture and subsequent compression following sheath removal can help prevent iatrogenic pseudoaneurysms.
- If suspected clinically, pseudoaneurysms can be easily diagnosed by color Doppler ultrasound.
- Ultrasound-guided thrombin injection is the treatment of choice for femoral pseudoaneurysms. It is quick, pain-free, safe, and reliable.
- Complications with thrombin injection leading to vessel thrombosis or distal embolization are rare and can be avoided by the use of small doses injected under continuous color Doppler ultrasound imaging.

- Pseudoaneurysms with short and wide necks can be treated using the same technique, but some operators prefer to place an occlusive balloon in the parent artery during thrombin injection.

Commentary

As a general rule, pseudoaneurysms smaller than 2 cm are likely to thrombose spontaneously and do not need to be treated unless they are symptomatic. The recommended "cut-off" in terms of pseudoaneurysm neck size for treatment by thrombin injection varies, and no absolute measurements can be given.

If the neck is felt to be very wide, balloon occlusion of the native vessel can be carried out to protect the parent artery and aid thrombosis of the aneurysm sac. In this case the contralateral femoral artery is punctured and a crossover sheath is placed and guidewire access obtained past the pseudoaneurysm. An appropriately sized angioplasty balloon is positioned across the neck of the pseudoaneurysm and inflated. With the balloon inflated, percutaneous thrombin injection of the pseudoaneurysm is performed using the standard technique as described above, until complete thrombosis is achieved. The balloon is deflated after 10 min and an angiogram performed. If there is persistent filling of the pseudoaneurysm, the process is repeated.

Further Reading

Morgan R, Belli A-M. Current treatment methods for postcatheterization pseudoaneurysms. J Vasc Interv Radiol. 2003;14:697–710.

Weinmann EE, Chayen D, Kobzantzev ZV, Zaretsky M, Bass A. Treatment of post-catheterisation false aneurysms: ultrasound-guided compression vs ultrasound-guided thrombin injection. Eur J Vasc Endovasc Surg. 2002;23:68–72.

Chapter 7
Superficial Femoral Artery Thrombosis Post-angioplasty

Robert P. Allison, Anna Maria Belli, Joo-Young Chun, Raymond Chung, Raj Das, Andrew England, Karen Flood, Marie-France Giroux, Richard G. McWilliams, Robert Morgan, Nik Papadakos, Jai V. Patel, Raf Patel, Uday Patel, Lakshmi Ratnam, Reddi Prasad Yadavali, and John Rose

Abstract This case reviews the different approaches to dealing with acute thrombosis following angioplasty. An example of a thrombolysis regimen is given in addition to technique for thromboaspiration.

Keywords Complications • Angioplasty • Thrombosis • Thrombolysis

---

R.P. Allison
Department of Interventional Radiology,
University Hospitals Southampton,
Southampton, Hampshire, UK

A.M. Belli
Department of Radiology, St. George's
Hospital and Medical School, Blackshaw
Road, London SW17 0RE, UK
e-mail: anna.belli@stgeorges.nhs.uk

J.-Y. Chun • R. Chung
R. Das • R. Morgan • N. Papadakos
Department of Radiology, St. George's
Hospital, London, UK

A. England
Department of Radiography, University
of Salford, Manchester, UK

K. Flood
Department of Vascular Radiology,
Leeds General Infirmary, Leeds, UK

M.-F. Giroux
Department of Radiology, CHUM-Centre
Hospitalier de l'Université de Montréal,
Montreal, QC, Canada

R.G. McWilliams
Department of Radiology, Royal Liverpool
University Hospital, Liverpool, UK

J.V. Patel
Department of Radiology, The Leeds Teaching
Hospitals NHS Trust, Leeds, West Yorkshire, UK

R. Patel
Department of Radiology,
The Leeds Teaching Hospitals NHS Trust,
Leeds, West Yorkshire, UK
e-mail: rafpatel@gmail.com

U. Patel
Department of Diagnostic Radiology,
St. George's Hospital and Medical School,
Blackshaw Road, SW17 0QT London, UK
e-mail: uday.patel@stgeorges.nhs.uk

L. Ratnam
Department of Radiology, St. George's
Hospital, Blackshaw Road, SW17 0QT London, UK
e-mail: lakshmi.ratnam@nhs.net

R.P. Yadavali
Department of Radiology, Aberdeen
Royal Infirmary, Aberdeen, UK

J. Rose
Department of Interventional Radiology,
Freeman Hospital, Newcastle Upon Tyne
Hospitals NHS Trust, Newcastle upon Tyne, UK

Case History

A morbidly obese 58-year-old male presented with rest pain in his left foot. His other relevant medical history was of insulin-dependent diabetes, hypertension, and hyperlipidemia. The patient was too large to be imaged in the departmental MRI scanner. A lower limb Doppler ultrasound examination demonstrated significant mid-left SFA stenosis, and angioplasty of this lesion was planned.

Procedure

The patient's body habitus and groin intertrigo precluded femoral access. Ultrasound-guided left brachial access was therefore used. Due to the patient's height, a 90 cm 4 Fr sheath only reached the aortic bifurcation. The longest 4 Fr catheter available at the time in the department, a 125 cm Berenstein catheter, only reached the common femoral artery. The focal stenotic lesion in the mid-SFA was visualized and luminally traversed with a 0.018″ guidewire (Fig. 7.1a). Luminal wire position was confirmed with contrast injection via the sheath. Following intra-arterial injection of 3,000 IU heparin, the only available balloon in the department that would reach the target lesion, a 4 mm × 20 cm angioplasty balloon, was inflated across the proximal/mid-SFA (Fig. 7.1b).

Check angiography following balloon deflation demonstrated de novo thrombosis of a segment of the angioplastied mid-SFA (Fig. 7.1c). The thrombus could not be reached by catheter or sheath for thromboaspiration. There was also no suitable stent available to reach the target. The patient was not considered a suitable candidate for surgery. The patient was given a further bolus of 5,000 IU heparin, and the thrombus was subsequently infused slowly with a total of 20 mg recombinant tissue plasminogen activator (rtPA) via the catheter in the SFA. The rtPA bolus resulted in restoration of

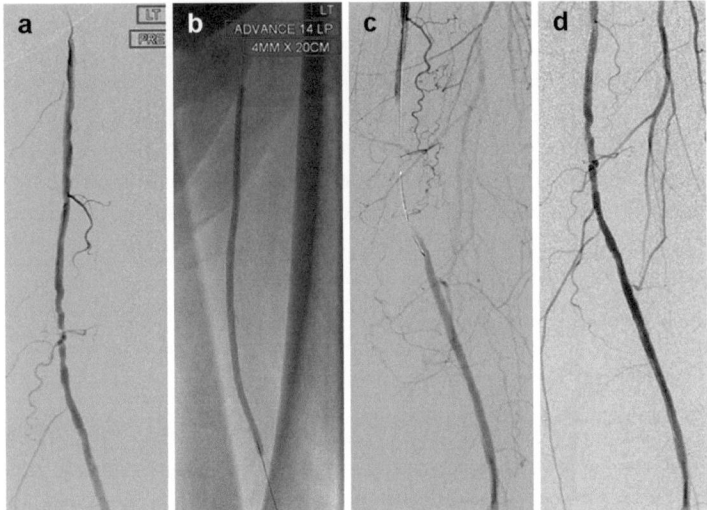

FIGURE 7.1 (**a**) Focal mid-SFA stenosis prior to angioplasty; (**b**) SFA angioplasty performed with a 4 mm × 20 cm balloon; (**c**) in situ SFA thrombosis following angioplasty which was flow-limiting; (**d**) restoration of satisfactory SFA flow following slowly titrated total dose of 10 mg tPA

flow to the SFA (Fig. 7.1d); however, the SFA thrombus migrated distally into the proximal crural arteries (Fig. 7.2a). The patient's foot was cool but viable. Following review and discussion with the attending vascular surgeon, the patient was commenced on a low-dose rtPA infusion (1 mg/h) to continue overnight, monitored on HDU. The following morning, 15 h after the start of the thrombolysis infusion, the patient returned for a check angiogram via the in situ catheter. This demonstrated the majority of thrombus in the crural arteries had cleared with significantly improved flow, two vessels crossing the ankle, and a warm well-perfused foot (Fig. 7.2b, c). A small volume of thrombus remained in the tibio-peroneal trunk but this was well collateralized. In view of the clinical improvement, the thrombolysis infusion was stopped. The patient made an uneventful recovery with an improvement in his left foot pain over the ensuing weeks.

Chapter 7. Superficial Femoral Artery Thrombosis

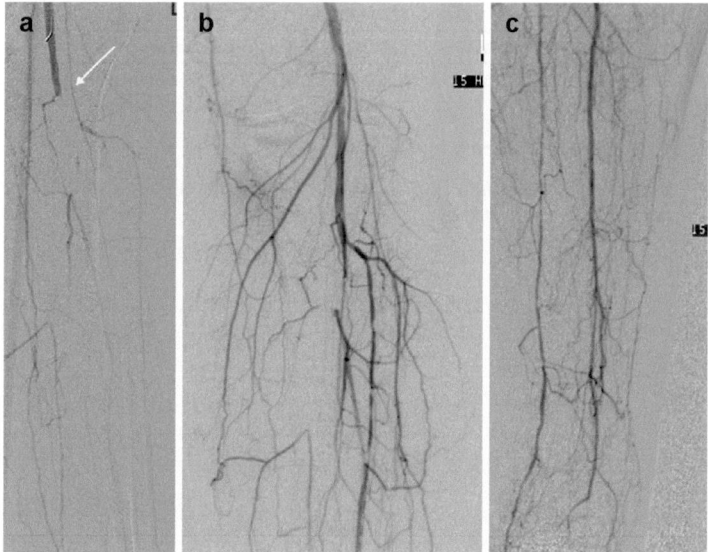

FIGURE 7.2 (**a**) Distal embolization of thrombus to calf vessels following initial tPA bolus (*arrow*); (**b**) restoration of satisfactory calf vessel flow following 15 h of tPA infusion (*Note*: there remains occlusive thrombus in the tibio-peroneal trunk); (**c**) satisfactory calf vessel flow following 15 h of tPA infusion with a PTA and ATA crossing the ankle. The foot was clinically well perfused at this stage and the tPA infusion was terminated

Discussion

Thrombosis following angioplasty is fortunately a rare event. If perfusion is critically impaired, endovascular treatment options include thrombolysis, thromboaspiration, angioplasty, and stenting. Surgical assistance should also be sought at an early stage as an alternative mode of treatment or if percutaneous methods fail. Alternatively, if a severely diseased and already narrowed artery becomes occluded, it may be of little clinical significance, especially if the limb distal to the occlusion remains perfused via collateral vessels. In this situation it may be appropriate not to pursue further invasive treatment.

TABLE 7.1 Absolute and relative contraindications to thrombolysis

Absolute contraindications	Relative contraindications
Active bleeding diathesis	Major surgery/trauma/cardiopulmonary resuscitation (within 2 weeks)
Recent gastrointestinal bleeding (within 2 weeks)	
Neurosurgery/intracranial trauma/hemorrhagic stroke (in the last 3 months)	Uncontrolled hypertension (systolic >180 mm Hg)
	Puncture of non-compressible vessel
	Recent eye surgery
	Diabetic retinopathy
	Hepatic failure
	Pregnancy

Recombinant tissue plasminogen activator (rtPA) is the most commonly used thrombolytic agent in the UK. In the presence of fibrin within thrombus, rtPA activates plasmin to break down the clot. Fresh thrombus is likely to respond well to thrombolysis.

While rtPA is relatively specific for thrombus, it should be remembered that thrombolysis, particularly with infusions, causes a systemic lytic state resulting in potential hemorrhagic complications. There are specific absolute and relative contraindications to be aware of (Table 7.1).

Small boluses of rtPA (5–10 mg) can be injected through a catheter directly into the thrombus. If this does not result in satisfactory dissolution of the thrombus, then an infusion of rtPA can be commenced through a catheter lodged in, or adjacent to, the thrombus. Various thrombolysis infusion dose regimes are described (usually between 0.25 and 2 mg rtPA per hour), with little evidence for superiority of any particular regime. It is best to be familiar with the one in use in your department.

If placed on a thrombolysis infusion, it is important the patient is monitored in a suitable environment such as a high dependency unit to identify any bleeding complications. Interval check angiography is performed every 6–18 h to assess progress and determine whether further thrombolysis is required. Infusions are not usually continued for more than 48 h.

Distal embolization of fragments of thrombus can occur during thrombolysis and can usually be treated with further rtPA or other endovascular or surgical techniques. Embolization of tiny fragments of thrombus may be more serious and can cause ischemic complications. Angioplasty and stenting may be required following thrombolysis if dissolution of the thrombus reveals an underlying lesion such as unstable plaque or a dissection.

Thromboaspiration is a useful technique and is frequently used as an adjunct to thrombolysis. A wide-bore catheter or long sheath is lodged in the thrombus, and suction is applied with a 50 ml syringe while the catheter is advanced to "suck" as much thrombus as possible. While maintaining suction the catheter is then withdrawn through an appropriately sized sheath with a removable hub. This technique can be repeated as required, but the main disadvantages are that wire access to the lesion is lost during catheter removal and also a larger arterial puncture site is required to allow a sufficiently sized sheath (usually 6–8 Fr). In the case described above, this technique could not be utilized as a catheter would not reach the thrombosed segment, and shorter routes of access were not possible.

Angioplasty and stenting are useful techniques to treat underlying causative lesions as well as prevent distal embolization, although the risk of embolization is not eliminated and further thrombus formation is possible. Surgical embolectomy should be considered if the thrombosis is in a critical vessel and resistant to percutaneous techniques or is complicated by distal embolization not amenable to endovascular treatment.

Tips

- Vessel thrombosis can be treated by a variety of endovascular techniques including thrombolysis, thromboaspiration, angioplasty, and stenting as well as surgical methods.
- Individual situations should determine the most appropriate course of intervention, if any, for post-angioplasty vessel thrombosis.
- Fresh thrombus responds most rapidly to thrombolysis and thromboaspiration.

- The interventionalist should be familiar with the range of emergency techniques which are often complimentary but are not without their own specific risks.
- Surgical advice should be sought early and the patient kept under close monitoring and review arrangements to ensure any deterioration or complication of treatment is detected swiftly and treated appropriately.

Commentary

As stated by the authors, there are various regimes available for administration of thrombolysis. It is our practice to administer a bolus of 5 mg (5 ml) of tPA via the catheter directly into thrombus. This is followed by an infusion of 0.5 mg/h of tPA – made up of 2.5 ml of tPA in 47.5 ml of normal saline which is then infused at a rate of 10 ml/h. It is important that an infusion of intravenous heparin is continued simultaneously.

There is no consensus on the method of delivering the thrombolysis. Although there are various infusion catheters and wires available, in our practice, a simple end-hole catheter is used via a 6 Fr vascular sheath and is placed within the thrombus. No advantage has been demonstrated in the literature of the use of multiple side-hole catheter versus end-hole only catheters. If there is some lysis of thrombus at the first check angiogram, the catheter is repositioned appropriately to tackle the residual thrombus.

It is important to ensure that the arterial puncture for access is a single puncture when the purpose is thrombolysis, and ultrasound guidance is helpful in achieving this to avoid bleeding via multiple attempted puncture sites when thrombolysis is commenced.

Further Reading

Cleveland TJ, Cumberland DC, Gaines PA. Percutaneous aspiration thromboembolectomy to manage the embolic complications of angioplasty and as an adjunct to thrombolysis. Clin Radiol. 1994;49:549–52.

Hall TB, Matson M, Belli AM. Thrombolysis in the peripheral vascular system. Eur Radiol. 2001;11:439–45.

Kessel DO, Berridge DC, Robertson I. Infusion techniques for peripheral arterial thrombolysis. Cochrane Database Syst Rev. 2004;2004(1):CD000985.

Morgan R, Belli AM. Percutaneous thrombectomy: a review. Eur Radiol. 2002;12:205–17.

Chapter 8
Superficial Femoral Artery Rupture Following Angioplasty

Robert P. Allison, Anna Maria Belli, Joo-Young Chun, Raymond Chung, Raj Das, Andrew England, Karen Flood, Marie-France Giroux, Richard G. McWilliams, Robert Morgan, Nik Papadakos, Jai V. Patel, Raf Patel, Uday Patel, Lakshmi Ratnam, Reddi Prasad Yadavali, and John Rose

Abstract This case reviews the various options for treating arterial rupture post-angioplasty including a discussion of principles to be adhered to in order to avoid such a situation in the first place.

Keywords Complications • Post-angioplasty • Rupture • Extravasation

---

R.P. Allison
Department of Interventional Radiology,
University Hospitals Southampton,
Southampton, Hampshire, UK

A.M. Belli
Department of Radiology, St. George's Hospital
and Medical School, Blackshaw Road,
London SW17 0RE, UK
e-mail: anna.belli@stgeorges.nhs.uk

J.-Y. Chun • R. Chung
R. Das • R. Morgan • N. Papadakos
Department of Radiology, St. George's
Hospital, London, UK

A. England
Department of Radiography, University
of Salford, Manchester, UK

K. Flood
Department of Vascular Radiology,
Leeds General Infirmary, Leeds, UK

M.-F. Giroux
Department of Radiology, CHUM-Centre
Hospitalier de l'Université de Montréal,
Montreal, QC, Canada

R.G. McWilliams
Department of Radiology, Royal Liverpool
University Hospital, Liverpool, UK

J.V. Patel
Department of Radiology, The Leeds Teaching
Hospitals NHS Trust, Leeds, West Yorkshire, UK

R. Patel
Department of Radiology, The Leeds Teaching
Hospitals NHS Trust, Leeds, West Yorkshire, UK
e-mail: rafpatel@gmail.com

U. Patel
Department of Diagnostic Radiology,
St. George's Hospital and Medical School,
Blackshaw Road, SW17 0QT London, UK
e-mail: uday.patel@stgeorges.nhs.uk

L. Ratnam
Department of Radiology, St. George's Hospital,
Blackshaw Road, SW17 0QT London, UK
e-mail: lakshmi.ratnam@nhs.net

R.P. Yadavali
Department of Radiology, Aberdeen Royal
Infirmary, Aberdeen, UK

J. Rose
Department of Interventional Radiology,
Freeman Hospital, Newcastle Upon Tyne
Hospitals NHS Trust, Newcastle upon Tyne, UK

Case History

A 68-year-old gentleman attended for right SFA angioplasty for recent onset short distance claudication. Past medical history included a prosthetic aortic valve, CABG, and TIA 10 years previously. The patient was on regular aspirin 75 mg OD and warfarin; the pre-procedural INR was 1.4 and hemoglobin and platelet count were normal.

Procedure

Arterial access was via a right CFA antegrade puncture and placement of a 6 Fr sheath, although insertion of the 6 Fr sheath was difficult due to soft tissue resistance. Angiograms demonstrated a 6 cm occlusion of the mid to distal SFA (Fig. 8.1a, b). Recanalization was successful via a subintimal passage because of the heavily calcified plaque.

Following angioplasty, there was extravasation of contrast from the angioplasty site (Fig. 8.2a). Balloon occlusion across the leak was successfully performed resulting in only minimal subsequent extravasation. Due to residual stenosis of the proximal portion of the plaque, an uncovered stent was inserted (Bard Luminexx −6×80 mm). At the end of the procedure, following stent placement, there remained minor extravasation extending approximately 1–2 cm around the site of rupture (Fig. 8.2b).

Placement of a covered stent/stent-graft was considered but would have required insertion of an 8 Fr antegrade sheath. Due to the difficulties with initial antegrade access, it was decided to avoid this and review the patient following overnight observation and an ultrasound duplex the following day. The duplex study demonstrated patent artery and no residual bleeding. No further intervention was required and the patient was discharged the following day.

Discussion

Vessel rupture is the most serious complication encountered following angioplasty. In the peripheral circulation this is usually self-limiting due to tamponade by the surrounding soft

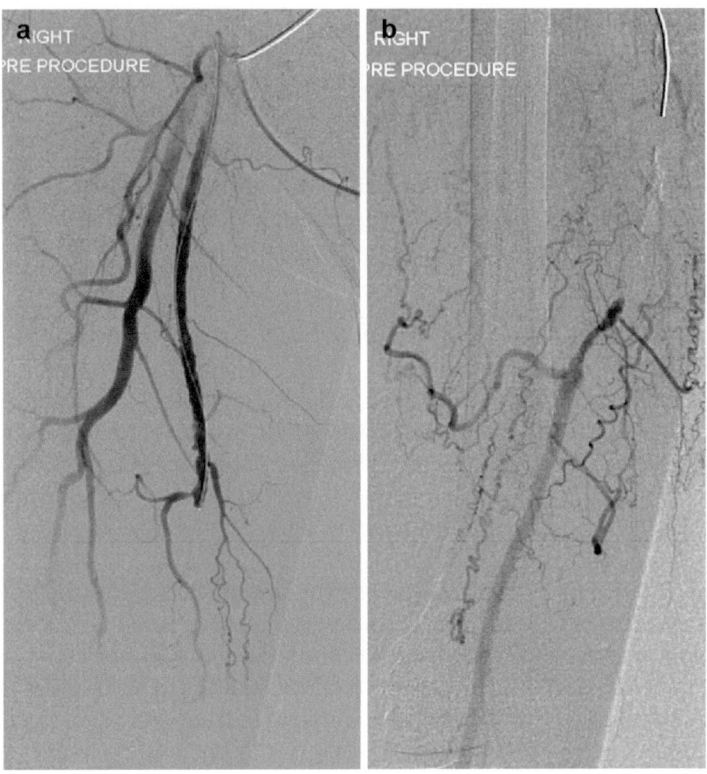

Figure 8.1 (**a**) Demonstrates right mid to (**b**) distal SFA occlusion

tissues; however, if in the thorax or abdomen, vessel rupture is usually life-threatening. Aside from angiographic evidence of contrast extravasation, clinical indicators of vessel rupture include severe pain experienced by the patient and hemodynamic deterioration.

If the vessel rupture is in the peripheral circulation and is minor, then conservative management may be all that is necessary. Immediate management of vessel rupture in the thorax or abdomen involves maintenance of guidewire access of the ruptured artery followed by immediate balloon reinflation across the extravasation site to control bleeding with subsequent placement of a stent-graft. Alternatively, embolization of the

Chapter 8. Superficial Femoral Artery Rupture 59

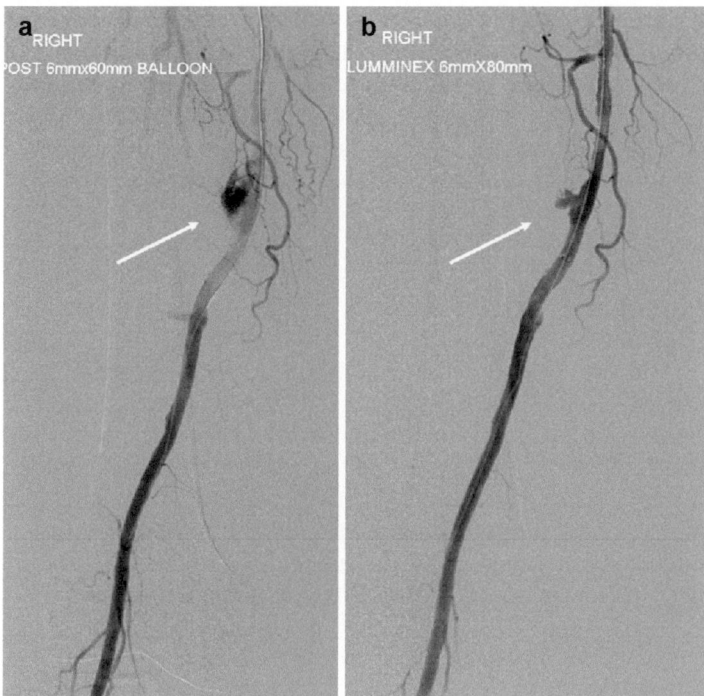

FIGURE 8.2 (**a**) Extravasation of contrast at the angioplasty site in the right SFA (*arrow*); (**b**) minor extravasation of contrast following bare metal stent deployment at the angioplasty site in the right SFA

artery can be performed followed by bypass surgery, or the patient may be transferred to theatre for surgical repair.

Rupture occurs more commonly due to eccentric calcified plaque at the angioplasty site, following use of a cutting balloon or high-pressure balloon angioplasty. Avoidance of vessel rupture is potentially aided by adhering to good principles of angioplasty. Most interventional radiologists choose angioplasty balloon diameters based on visual estimation. If in doubt, use of a balloon of smaller diameter with an accurate roadmap is recommended, and if the balloon is too small, then repeat angioplasty with a larger one can be performed subsequently.

Attention to the angioplasty balloon manufacturer's recommendations is important. The nominal pressure is the pressure at which the balloon reaches its rated diameter. The burst pressure is the average pressure that is required to rupture the balloon. The rated burst pressure is the highest pressure to which the balloon can be inflated with minimal chance of bursting. Use of a pressure inflation device allows more accurate inflation to the recommended pressures. The case described above also illustrates that vessel rupture or extravasation in the peripheral arteries does not necessarily require stent-graft insertion.

The use of covered stents traditionally requires a large sheath, usually greater than 8 Fr. Newer developments in stent-graft technology mean that 6 or 7 Fr sheaths can be used for the SFA or other vessels of the order of 6–7 mm diameter. Examples are the Gore® Viabahn® and Atrium™ Advanta V12 covered stents. With familiarity and knowledge of different techniques and available stent-grafts operators can usually deal with most vessel ruptures by endovascular means.

Commentary

As illustrated by the case above, arterial rupture does not always require placement of a stent-graft in the peripheral circulation and often responds to conservative measures. Rupture as a result of extraluminal recanalization during angioplasty is often self-limiting. When performing subintimal angioplasty, it is crucial to confirm that you are back in the true lumen of the parent vessel and not in a branch vessel before performing balloon dilatation. Rupture of a branch vessel is less likely to be self-limiting. In such a situation, prolonged balloon dilatation (5–10 min) across the origin of the branch vessel should be performed. If the bleeding does not stop and the vessel can be occluded, coil embolization of the vessel can be performed which will stop the bleeding.

When performing angioplasty, in particular within the thorax and abdomen, it is good practice to ensure that an appropriate size stent-graft and sheath are available in the interventional room at the beginning of the procedure. Should there be a vessel rupture, this minimizes time taken to proceed to appropriate endovascular treatment. Many units have a "rupture box" containing the appropriate equipment, primarily for dealing with iliac ruptures.

Further Reading

Tsetis D. Endovascular treatment of complications of femoral arterial access. Cardiovasc Intervent Radiol. 2010;33(3):457–68.

Chapter 9
Distal Embolization Following Common Iliac and Superficial Femoral Artery Angioplasty

Robert P. Allison, Anna Maria Belli, Joo-Young Chun, Raymond Chung, Raj Das, Andrew England, Karen Flood, Marie-France Giroux, Richard G. McWilliams, Robert Morgan, Nik Papadakos, Jai V. Patel, Raf Patel, Uday Patel, Lakshmi Ratnam, Reddi Prasad Yadavali, and John Rose

Abstract This case discusses the complication of distal embolization following angioplasty. Management of distal embolization from thromboaspiration to thrombolysis is also reviewed.

Keywords Complications • Post-angioplasty • Distal embolization

---

R.P. Allison
Department of Interventional Radiology,
University Hospitals Southampton,
Southampton, Hampshire, UK

A.M. Belli
Department of Radiology, St. George's
Hospital and Medical School, Blackshaw
Road, London SW17 0RE, UK
e-mail: anna.belli@stgeorges.nhs.uk

J.-Y. Chun • R. Chung
R. Das • R. Morgan • N. Papadakos
Department of Radiology, St. George's Hospital, London, UK

A. England
Department of Radiography, University of Salford, Manchester, UK

K. Flood
Department of Vascular Radiology,
Leeds General Infirmary, Leeds, UK

M.-F. Giroux
Department of Radiology, CHUM-Centre
Hospitalier de l'Université de Montréal,
Montreal, QC, Canada

R.G. McWilliams
Department of Radiology, Royal Liverpool
University Hospital, Liverpool, UK

J.V. Patel
Department of Radiology, The Leeds Teaching
Hospitals NHS Trust, Leeds, West Yorkshire, UK

R. Patel
Department of Radiology,
The Leeds Teaching Hospitals NHS Trust,
Leeds, West Yorkshire, UK
e-mail: rafpatel@gmail.com

U. Patel
Department of Diagnostic Radiology,
St. George's Hospital and Medical School,
Blackshaw Road, SW17 0QT London, UK
e-mail: uday.patel@stgeorges.nhs.uk

L. Ratnam
Department of Radiology, St. George's Hospital,
Blackshaw Road, SW17 0QT London, UK
e-mail: lakshmi.ratnam@nhs.net

R.P. Yadavali
Department of Radiology, Aberdeen Royal
Infirmary, Aberdeen, UK

J. Rose
Department of Interventional Radiology,
Freeman Hospital, Newcastle Upon Tyne
Hospitals NHS Trust, Newcastle upon Tyne, UK

Chapter 9. Distal Embolization Post Angioplasty   65

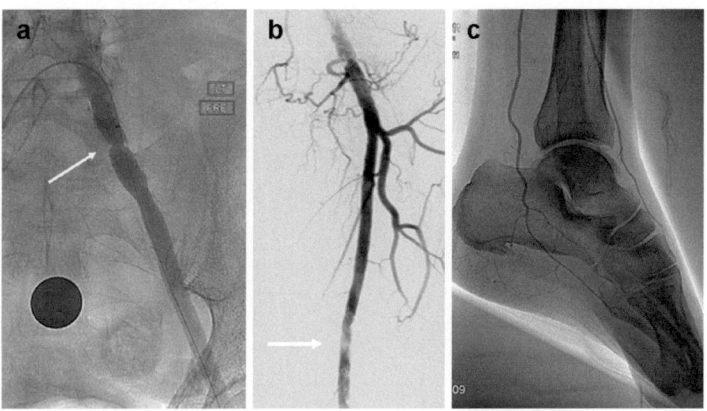

FIGURE 9.1 (a) Angiography demonstrating weblike left CIA stenosis (*arrow*); (b) calcified left SFA stenosis (*arrow*); (c) good plantar flow seen pre-angioplasty

Case History

A 67-year-old man presented with left foot rest pain and blue toes. A diagnosis of blue toe syndrome was confirmed on magnetic resonance angiography (MRA) where stenoses of the left common iliac (CIA) and superficial femoral arteries (SFA) were identified as potential sources of emboli.

Procedure

A retrograde puncture of the right common femoral artery (CFA) was performed, and a 5 Fr 45cm-long sheath was placed over the bifurcation. Angiography demonstrated weblike stenoses of the left CIA (Fig. 9.1a) and significant calcified stenoses in the mid SFA (Fig. 9.1b), with 3-vessel runoff in the calf and good plantar flow (Fig. 9.1c). Angioplasty was performed to remodel the stenoses using a 10 mm balloon in the CIA and 6 mm in the SFA. A good post-angioplasty result was seen. However, slow flow was identified in the left posterior tibial artery (PT), with

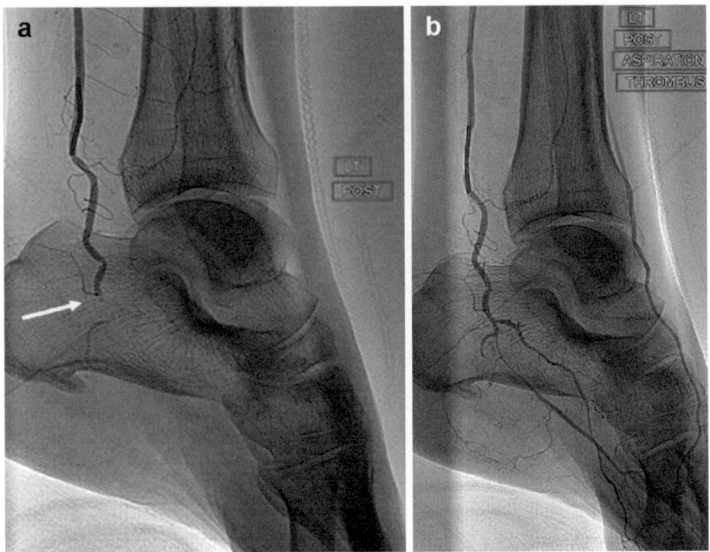

FIGURE 9.2 (**a**) Occlusive thrombus in PT behind malleolus causing abrupt cessation of flow (*arrow*); (**b**) angiography post-thromboaspiration demonstrating restored PT and plantar flow

occlusive thrombus in this vessel behind the medial malleolus (Fig. 9.2a).

Catheters were not long enough to reach the distal embolus via the right groin puncture. An ultrasound-guided antegrade left CFA puncture was performed, and a 5 Fr 55-cm sheath was inserted into the proximal posterior tibial artery. A bolus of antispasmodics was given (150-mcg GTN). Thromboaspiration was performed with two passes in the PT and plantar artery using a 5 Fr Berenstein catheter inserted through the sheath (this is important as you are not likely to put anything much larger in this site!) with successful removal of thrombus. Completion angiography demonstrated restored PT and plantar flow (Fig. 9.2b).

Discussion

Embolization occurs in 3–7 % of patients post-iliac angioplasty and is more common in occlusive disease. The nature of emboli (plaque, thrombus, or cholesterol) determines the success of the different therapeutic options.

If distal embolization occurs, good-quality angiograms are required to assess the runoff and presence of collateral vessels. Clinical assessment of the limb is important. If the limb is well perfused and the embolus is in a non-critical branch, then further intervention is inappropriate. If, as in this case, the embolus is sitting in a major vessel, then treatment is required to restore blood flow distally.

Clot aspiration is performed using the largest bore catheter that can be safely used in the territory and a sheath with a detachable hub. The aspiration catheter is embedded into the proximal occlusion and a 50-ml syringe attached. The syringe plunger is pulled back to create a vacuum, and the catheter is advanced into the thrombus with suction maintained; the catheter is then withdrawn. As the catheter reaches the sheath, the hub is removed to prevent trapping thrombus on the hemostatic valve as the catheter is removed. The contents of the catheter and syringe should be flushed through a gauze cloth to allow examination. This can be repeated as often as necessary until the vessel is clear.

Although not done in this case, as clot aspiration was successful, balloon maceration of thrombus +/− local thrombolysis can be given. However, local thrombolytic infusion may work poorly if the embolus is solid material, e.g., plaque.

Tips

- Distal embolization is a recognized complication of angioplasty.
- Good-quality angiography is necessary to identify the level of the embolus.

- Emboli in major vessels can be removed using the technique of thromboaspiration.
- Local thrombolysis can be used to dissolve the embolic material, although success is less likely if the emboli are secondary to solid material, e.g., plaque.
- Occasionally large emboli have to be surgically removed.

Commentary

Distal embolization is a well-recognized complication of angioplasty. Angiography of the runoff pre- and post-angioplasty should be performed in order to be aware if this has occurred so appropriate treatment can be undertaken. When performing angioplasty or stenting of proximal common iliac artery occlusions or stenoses, a kissing balloon/stent technique may be employed to prevent embolus from passing down the contralateral limb. Primary stenting of iliac occlusions without initial angioplasty should also be performed to reduce the risk of distal embolization.

For details on performing thrombolysis, see discussion and commentary on case 7 (SFA thrombosis post-angioplasty, Chap. 7).

Further Reading

British Society of Interventional Iliac Angioplasty Study (BIAS). Oxfordshire Dendrite Clinical Systems; 2001. ISBN 1-903968-01-1; http://www.bsir.org

Chapter 10
Flow-Limiting Iliac Artery Dissection Post-angioplasty

Robert P. Allison, Anna Maria Belli, Joo-Young Chun, Raymond Chung, Raj Das, Andrew England, Karen Flood, Marie-France Giroux, Richard G. McWilliams, Robert Morgan, Nik Papadakos, Jai V. Patel, Raf Patel, Uday Patel, Lakshmi Ratnam, Reddi Prasad Yadavali, and John Rose

Abstract This case discusses when and how to treat a post-angioplasty arterial dissection. The merits of balloon expanding and self-expanding stents are also discussed.

Keywords Complications • Post-angioplasty • Arterial dissection

---

R.P. Allison
Department of Interventional Radiology,
University Hospitals Southampton, Southampton, Hampshire, UK

A.M. Belli
Department of Radiology, St. George's Hospital and Medical School,
Blackshaw Road, London SW17 0RE, UK
e-mail: anna.belli@stgeorges.nhs.uk

J.-Y. Chun • R. Chung • R. Das
R. Morgan • N. Papadakos
Department of Radiology, St. George's Hospital, London, UK

A. England
Department of Radiography, University of Salford, Manchester, UK

K. Flood
Department of Vascular Radiology, Leeds General Infirmary,
Leeds, UK

M.-F. Giroux
Department of Radiology, CHUM-Centre Hospitalier
de l'Université de Montréal, Montreal, QC, Canada

R.G. McWilliams
Department of Radiology, Royal Liverpool University Hospital,
Liverpool, UK

J.V. Patel
Department of Radiology, The Leeds Teaching Hospitals NHS Trust,
Leeds, West Yorkshire, UK

R. Patel
Department of Radiology,
The Leeds Teaching Hospitals NHS Trust,
Leeds, West Yorkshire, UK
e-mail: rafpatel@gmail.com

U. Patel
Department of Radiology, St. George's Hospital and Medical School,
Blackshaw Road, SW17 0QT London, UK
e-mail: uday.patel@stgeorges.nhs.uk

L. Ratnam
Department of Radiology, St. George's Hospital, Blackshaw Road,
SW17 0QT London, UK
e-mail: lakshmi.ratnam@nhs.net

R.P. Yadavali
Department of Radiology, Aberdeen Royal Infirmary, Aberdeen, UK

J. Rose
Department of Interventional Radiology, Freeman Hospital,
Newcastle Upon Tyne Hospitals NHS Trust, Newcastle upon Tyne, UK

Chapter 10. Arterial Dissection Post-angioplasty

Case History

A 52-year-old gentleman presented with 100 m left leg claudication. Magnetic resonance angiography (MRA) demonstrated stenoses of the mid-left common iliac and origin of the external iliac artery. He was brought into the department for a day case angioplasty procedure.

Procedure

A retrograde puncture of the left common femoral artery was performed, with placement of a 4 Fr sheath. Three thousand units of heparin were given via the sheath, and a Terumo wire and Cobra catheter were used to cross the stenoses. AP and oblique left iliac artery angiography was performed after administration of 20 mg Buscopan. The common (CIA) and external iliac artery (EIA) stenoses were confirmed (Fig. 10.1a). Angioplasty of these regions was performed using an 8 × 40 mm low-profile balloon. Completion angiography demonstrated a

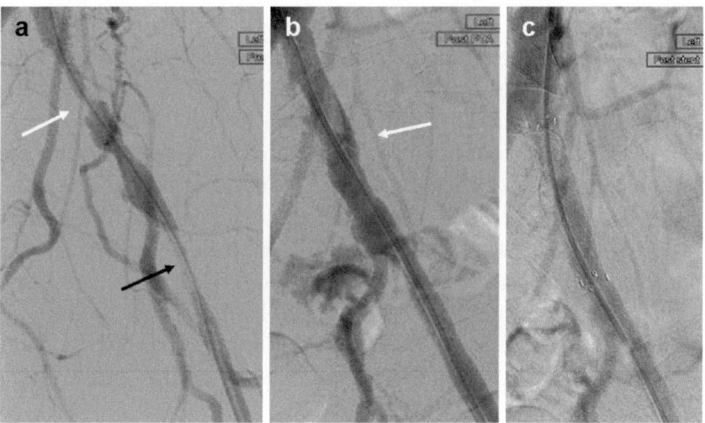

FIGURE 10.1 (**a**) Angiography demonstrating left CIA (*white arrow*) and EIA stenoses (*black arrow*); (**b**) dissection flap seen in left CIA (*arrow*); (**c**) CIA stent, with good flow

dissection flap within the common iliac artery, which was flow-limiting causing >50 % luminal narrowing (Fig. 10.1b).

The 4 Fr sheath was exchanged for a 6 Fr sheath, and secondary stenting, using an 8 × 40 mm self-expanding stent, was performed to treat and pin back the left CIA dissection flap (Fig. 10.1c). Good flow was seen following this, with three vessel runoff in the calf.

Discussion

In the case of iliac stenotic disease, angioplasty (PTA) is the procedure of choice. Stenting is indicated when there is a >30 % residual stenosis, a residual peak systolic gradient of >10 mm Hg, or a flow-limiting dissection. The aim of stenting is to eliminate or reduce the dissection flap and to restore luminal patency to a size commensurate with the diameter of the vessel segments above and below the stent. In this case the dissection flap was flow-limiting and causing a >50 % reduction in lumen size. Prolonged balloon inflation could have been attempted to reduce the dissection flap without stenting, but due to its extent, stenting was felt to be a better option.

Primary stent placement is generally accepted in clinical practice for patients with chronic iliac artery occlusions and with recurrent stenosis after previous iliac PTA, though there is still little evidence to support the latter approach.

Appropriate stent choice depends on the lesion morphology and location. When dealing with lesions of high elastic recoil, such as calcified or eccentric plaques at the ostium of the CIA or EIA, a balloon-expanded stent is more appropriate than a self-expanding due to greater resistance to extrinsic compression. A self-expanding stent should be chosen to stabilize longer, less calcified vessel segments. In this case a self-expanding stent was used, to exert some additional force on the dissection flap.

Tips

- Flow-limiting dissections/elastic recoil of the artery post-angioplasty should be treated with prolonged balloon inflation +/− secondary stenting.

- The aim of the treatment is to eliminate or reduce the dissection flap and restore luminal flow.
- If approaching from the contralateral groin, a long sheath over the bifurcation may provide added support when deploying a stent.
- Balloon-expanded stents are recommended for heavily calcified lesions, as they offer more radial force.

Commentary

Before commencing angioplasty of the iliac arteries, you should always ensure the availability of both bare and covered stents in case of either a dissection, inadequate angioplasty result, or an arterial rupture.

Arterial dissections are a direct consequence of angioplasty but may also occur as a result of guidewire trauma at the time of crossing a stenosis or occlusion. If a dissection occurs against the flow of blood (e.g., in the case of a retrograde CFA puncture), it is likely to be self-limiting as the force of the blood flow in the opposite direction will often close the flap. If it occurs in the direction of blood flow, then it is likely to become flow-limiting as the flap is kept open by the direction of blood flowing from the aorta. It is important to obtain through and through luminal communication across the dissected segment before proceeding to prolonged balloon dilatation or stenting.

Further Reading

Quality Improvement Guidelines for Endovascular Treatment of Iliac Artery Occlusive Disease. CIRSE: http://cirse.org/. Accessed 11 Apr 2013.

Tetteroo E, Haaring C, van der Graaf Y, van Schaik JP, van Engelen AD, Mali WP. Intraarterial pressure gradients after randomized angioplasty or stenting of iliac artery lesions. Dutch Iliac Stent Trial Study Group. Cardiovasc Intervent Radiol. 1996;19(6):411–7.

Vorwerk D, Gunther RW. Percutaneous interventions for treatment of iliac artery stenoses and occlusions. World J Surg. 2001;25:319–27.

Chapter 11
Dissection of Superior Mesenteric Artery (SMA) During Transarterial Chemoembolization (TACE) via a Replaced Right Hepatic Artery

Robert P. Allison, Anna Maria Belli, Joo-Young Chun, Raymond Chung, Raj Das, Andrew England, Karen Flood, Marie-France Giroux, Richard G. McWilliams, Robert Morgan, Nik Papadakos, Jai V. Patel, Raf Patel, Uday Patel, Lakshmi Ratnam, Reddi Prasad Yadavali, and John Rose

Abstract This case describes dissection of the origin of the SMA during cannulation for transarterial chemoembolization (TACE) procedure. Techniques to overcome this situation and restore flow are discussed as well as schematic diagrams illustrating the flow dynamics in a dissection.

Keywords Complications • Embolization • Dissection • Transarterial chemoembolization (TACE)

R.P. Allison
Department of Interventional Radiology, University Hospitals Southampton, Southampton, Hampshire, UK

A.M. Belli
Department of Radiology, St. George's Hospital and Medical
School, Blackshaw Road, London SW17 0RE, UK
e-mail: anna.belli@stgeorges.nhs.uk

J.-Y. Chun • R. Chung • R. Das
R. Morgan • N. Papadakos
Department of Radiology, St. George's Hospital, London, UK

A. England
Department of Radiography, University of Salford, Manchester, UK

K. Flood
Department of Vascular Radiology, Leeds General Infirmary,
Leeds, UK

M.-F. Giroux
Department of Radiology, CHUM-Centre Hospitalier de
l'Université de Montréal, Montreal, QC, Canada

R.G. McWilliams
Department of Radiology, Royal Liverpool University Hospital,
Liverpool, UK

J.V. Patel
Department of Radiology, The Leeds Teaching Hospitals
NHS Trust, Leeds, West Yorkshire, UK

R. Patel
Department of Radiology,
The Leeds Teaching Hospitals NHS Trust,
Leeds, West Yorkshire, UK
e-mail: rafpatel@gmail.com

U. Patel
Department of Radiology, St. George's Hospital
and Medical School, Blackshaw Road, SW17 0QT London, UK
e-mail: uday.patel@stgeorges.nhs.uk

L. Ratnam
Department of Radiology, St. George's Hospital,
Blackshaw Road, SW17 0QT London, UK
e-mail: lakshmi.ratnam@nhs.net

R.P. Yadavali
Department of Radiology, Aberdeen Royal Infirmary,
Aberdeen, UK

J. Rose
Department of Interventional Radiology, Freeman Hospital,
Newcastle Upon Tyne Hospitals NHS Trust,
Newcastle upon Tyne, UK

Case History

A 57-year-old man was found to have a 5 cm hepatocellular carcinoma during investigations for hepatitis C. He had no history of alcohol abuse but smoked 10 cigarettes/day. He was asymptomatic at the time of referral for treatment of the HCC with normal performance status. Apart from a slight increase in transaminase levels his LFTs were normal. Alpha fetoprotein was elevated at 1,129 u. CT scan performed prior to the procedure demonstrated a posterior right hepatic tumor (segment 7) and also demonstrated that the right hepatic artery is replaced from the SMA and thus lies in the portacaval space.

Procedure

Following standard Seldinger access through the right common femoral artery with placement of a 5 Fr vascular sheath, a Sidewinder 2 catheter was used to select the coeliac axis, and this confirmed that the left hepatic artery arose in isolation from the common hepatic trunk and did not give any obvious contribution to the right-sided tumor. The Sidewinder catheter was then placed in the ostium of the SMA, and this confirmed the position of the origin of the right hepatic artery (RHA) about 2 cm distally and arising at an acute angle from the SMA trunk. A soft-tipped guide wire (Bentson) was inserted down the main trunk and the Sidewinder pulled down in order to send the tip of the catheter further down the SMA. On retracting the catheter the tip would then normally move upward along the right wall of the SMA and fall into the RHA origin. This maneuver failed, and having repositioned the Sidewinder, gentle probing with a soft Terumo hydrophilic guide wire also failed to gain access to the RHA.

At this stage, the Sidewinder was exchanged for a Sos Omni catheter, and Fig. 11.1a shows the appearance of the RHA origin. This closer view of the origin appears to show that the origin is kinked and the angle with the SMA is more obtuse than acute, perhaps explaining the difficulty of

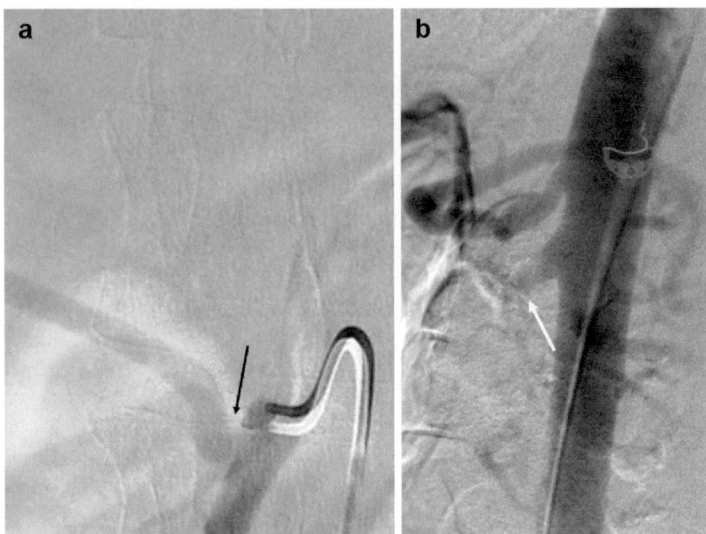

FIGURE 11.1 (**a**) Dissection of SMA origin (*arrow*) seen on selective imaging with Sos Omni; (**b**) confirmed on lateral aortogram via pigtail catheter (*arrow*)

catheterization with a reverse curve catheter. The image also shows a small dissection flap (arrow) adjacent to the catheter tip although no contrast was retained in this area after the injection ceased. The Sos catheter was exchanged (in the aorta) for a Cobra in order to produce a better angle of approach to the RHA ostium. At this stage there was reduced contrast opacification of the SMA main trunk, and it was clear that a flow-limiting dissection had been created.

The diagnosis of this complication was confirmed with a lateral pigtail aortogram (Fig. 11.1b), and the situation explained to the patient. Over the course of several minutes, the patient became increasingly symptomatic, with colicky abdominal pain and nausea. After administration of IV fentanyl and ondansetron, restoration of normal flow to the SMA was undertaken.

Chapter 11. Dissection of Superior Mesenteric Artery 79

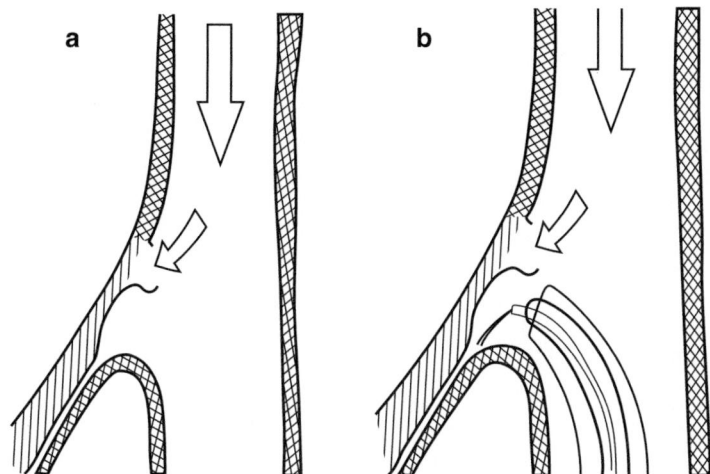

FIGURE 11.2 (**a**) SMA dissection flap held open by direction of flow (*arrows*) occluding the native vessel; (**b**) coaxial system of 6 Fr sheath, 4 Fr Cobra, and 2.6 Fr microcatheter (Progreat) used to access the collapsed lumen of the SMA

Bailout Procedure

Initial attempts to pass a hydrophilic 0.035″. Terumo wire beyond the dissection flap using the Cobra catheter seemed to make the dissection worse with the wire continually looping back. Therefore, the access sheath was upsized to 6 Fr, and a renal double curve guiding catheter inserted to the level of the SMA origin. A 4 Fr Cobra catheter was placed within the ostium of the SMA and rotated carefully while probing the area of the dissection flap with a coaxial Terumo Progreat and standard 0.018″ wire (Fig. 11.2a, b).

This was successful, but once the Progreat had been advanced to the patent lumen beyond the dissection, it was clear that the Cobra could not simply be railroaded along the Progreat and standard 0.018″ wire. Thus a more robust 0.014″ exchange wire (Stabilizer Plus, Cordis Endovascular, J&J, Berkshire, UK) was passed into a distal SMA branch, and this allowed

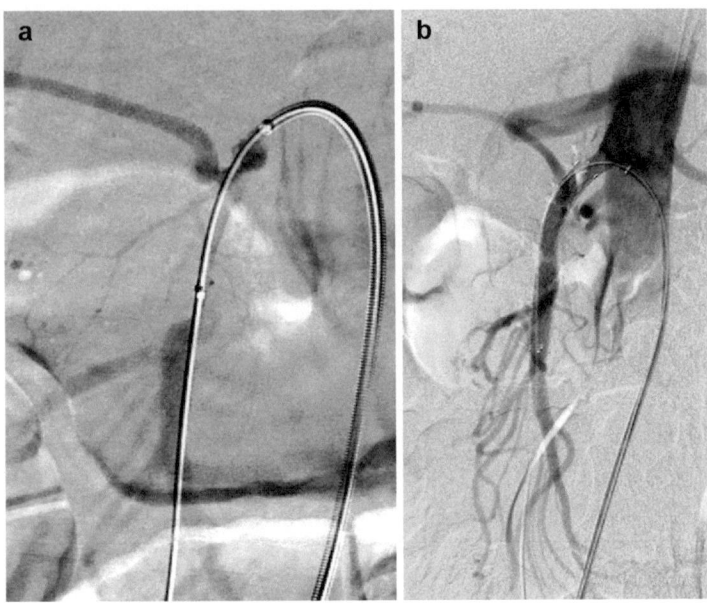

Figure 11.3 (**a**) Stiff guide wire allows passage of guiding sheath; (**b**) post-stent deployment

the gradual passage of the Cobra and the insertion of a stiff 0.035″ exchange wire (Fig. 11.3a).

Having secured access with a long Amplatz wire, the guiding catheter could then be advanced through the area of the dissection. An 8 mm diameter self-expanding stent (Luminexx, BARD UK) was then placed to scaffold the dissection flap (Fig. 11.3b).

The patient was discharged at 48 h on antiplatelet agents and an early CT follow-up confirmed patency of the SMA stent. Unfortunately chemoembolization will no longer be possible through the RHA, but the tumor should be accessible to percutaneous thermal ablation.

Discussion

Spasm and minor dissections of the hepatic artery are uncommon complications during chemoembolization procedures (1–2 %) and are generally self-limiting. In most cases the procedure can be halted while antispasmodics are administered, and in more severe cases, the procedure can be postponed and successfully completed at a later date. In this case a flow-limiting dissection occurred and this is an extremely rare event in the authors' experience. This might have been avoided by a more thorough inspection of the angle of origin of the RHA from the SMA on the preoperative CT and selection of a more appropriate catheter shape.

Clearly the main aim in dealing with a complication of this severity must be to restore blood flow to the gut swiftly, preferably by endovascular means. The SMA may be more reliably recanalized using an antegrade approach through brachial artery access. However, if a stable guiding catheter position can be achieved, as in this case, then modern small vessel catheters and fine caliber wires may be negotiated through the collapsed true lumen and into the more normal distal lumen. Long, robust 0.014″ exchange wires as used in carotid work may be very useful in this regard.

Tips

- Remember to gain as much anatomical information as possible prior to chemoembolization by careful inspection of the preoperative imaging.
- If there is any doubt about the origin of a hepatic vessel from the main trunk, then additional semi-selective angiography should be undertaken before super selecting the vessel.
- Sidewinder (Simmons) and Sos catheters are generally good for selecting acutely angled branch ostia.
- Cobra-type shapes are often safer for more obtuse angles.
- Beware the wire that loops soon after entering the lumen of a large vessel as a dissection space may have been created.

Commentary

Arterial dissection in the process of TACE is usually self-limiting and resolves spontaneously. Acute mesenteric ischemia secondary to arterial dissection may clinically manifest as abdominal pain, nausea, hemobilia, or jaundice. Delayed presentation can be due to pseudoaneurysm formation secondary to a dissection.

An acute dissection does not necessarily preclude proceeding with an embolization as planned although this may have to be performed by advancing a microcatheter past the dissected section of artery to achieve suitable position to proceed with embolization. The key to whether definitive treatment is required is if the dissection is flow limiting (illustrated by the line drawing) as was the case in the example above.

The use of a bare-metal stent and not a stent graft allows treatment of the dissection flap while preserving important side branches of the proximal SMA. Successful angioplasty of iatrogenic mesenteric arterial dissection flaps has also been described.

Further Reading

Lee K-H, Sung K-B, Lee D-Y, et al. Transcatheter arterial chemoembolisation for hepatocellular carcinoma: anatomic and haemodynamic considerations in the hepatic artery and portal vein. Radiographics. 2002;22:1077–91.

Sakamoto I, Aso N, Nagaoki K, et al. Complications associated with transcatheter arterial embolisation for hepatic tumours. Radiographics. 1998;18:605–19.

Chapter 12
Iatrogenic Iliac Artery Rupture During Arterial Stenting

Robert P. Allison, Anna Maria Belli, Joo-Young Chun, Raymond Chung, Raj Das, Andrew England, Karen Flood, Marie-France Giroux, Richard G. McWilliams, Robert Morgan, Nik Papadakos, Jai V. Patel, Raf Patel, Uday Patel, Lakshmi Ratnam, Reddi Prasad Yadavali, and John Rose

Abstract This case illustrates an example of iliac artery rupture, management measures to deal with this, and steps which can be taken to facilitate treatment to reduce risk to the patient should this happen.

Keywords Complications • Iliac angioplasty • Rupture • Stent graft

---

R.P. Allison
Department of Interventional Radiology, University Hospitals Southampton, Southampton, Hampshire, UK

A.M. Belli
Department of Radiology, St. George's Hospital and Medical School, Blackshaw Road, London SW17 0RE, UK
e-mail: anna.belli@stgeorges.nhs.uk

J.-Y. Chun • R. Chung • R. Das
R. Morgan • N. Papadakos
Department of Radiology, St. George's Hospital, London, UK

A. England
Department of Radiography, University of Salford,
Manchester, UK

K. Flood
Department of Vascular Radiology, Leeds General Infirmary,
Leeds, UK

M.-F. Giroux
Department of Radiology, CHUM-Centre Hospitalier de
l'Université de Montréal, Montreal, QC, Canada

R.G. McWilliams
Department of Radiology, Royal Liverpool University Hospital,
Liverpool, UK

J.V. Patel
Department of Radiology, The Leeds Teaching Hospitals
NHS Trust, Leeds, West Yorkshire, UK

R. Patel
Department of Radiology,
The Leeds Teaching Hospitals NHS Trust,
Leeds, West Yorkshire, UK
e-mail: rafpatel@gmail.com

U. Patel
Department of Diagnostic Radiology, St. George's Hospital
and Medical School, Blackshaw Road, SW17 0QT London, UK
e-mail: uday.patel@stgeorges.nhs.uk

L. Ratnam
Department of Radiology, St. George's Hospital, Blackshaw Road,
SW17 0QT London, UK
e-mail: lakshmi.ratnam@nhs.net

R.P. Yadavali
Department of Radiology, Aberdeen Royal Infirmary,
Aberdeen, UK

J. Rose
Department of Interventional Radiology, Freeman Hospital,
Newcastle Upon Tyne Hospitals NHS Trust,
Newcastle upon Tyne, UK

Chapter 12. Iatrogenic Iliac Artery Rupture 85

Case History

A 46-year-old female presented with left leg claudication secondary to a left iliac artery occlusion (Fig. 12.1a). Iliac recanalization and stenting was performed from a contralateral (right femoral) approach, over the aortic bifurcation. Two 7 mm diameter self-expanding stents were placed across the occlusion, and these were subsequently dilated with a 6 mm angioplasty balloon. At this point the patient experienced severe pain and became profoundly hypotensive. Angiography showed rupture of the external iliac artery (Fig. 12.1b).

Procedure

The angioplasty balloon was reinflated across the site of rupture (Fig. 12.2a) and the patient resuscitated. The left femoral artery was punctured under ultrasound guidance and a

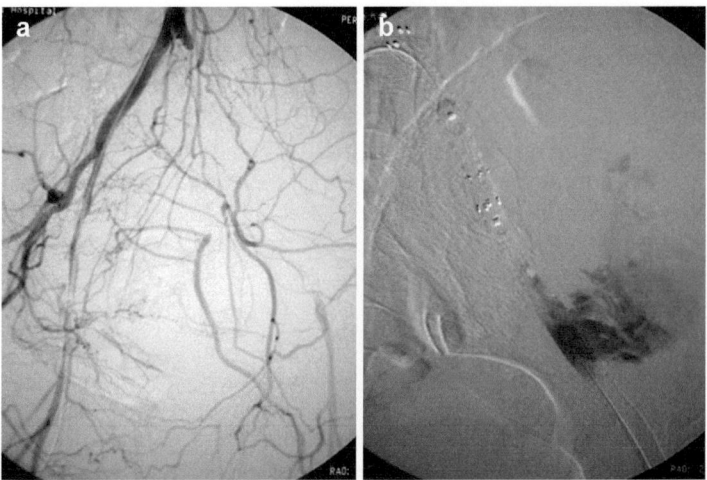

FIGURE 12.1 (a) Angiogram from a right femoral approach demonstrating occlusion of the left common and external iliac arteries; (b) angiogram confirming rupture of the left external iliac artery

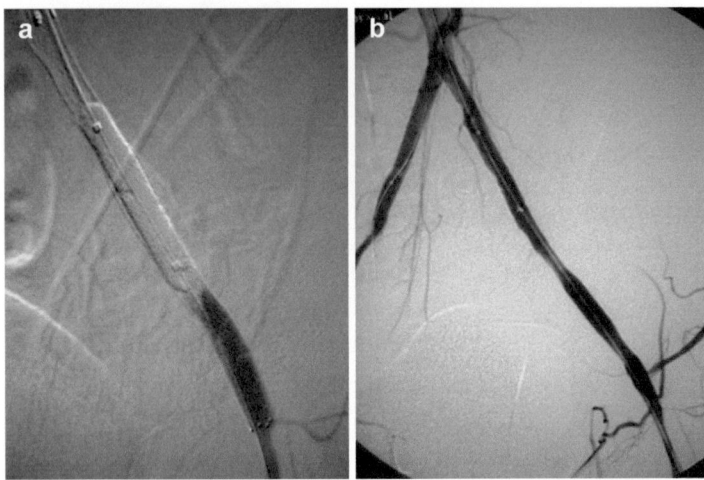

FIGURE 12.2 (**a**) The angioplasty balloon has been inflated across the site of rupture to provide temporary "hemostasis"; (**b**) the rupture has been sealed by placement of a balloon expandable stent graft

sheath placed. A Terumo guide wire and Cobra 2 catheter were negotiated past the inflated angioplasty balloon. These were exchanged for a super stiff Amplatz guide wire. A balloon expandable stent graft was passed into position while deflating the angioplasty balloon. The angioplasty balloon was withdrawn and the stent graft rapidly deployed to seal the rupture (Fig. 12.2b).

Discussion

Arterial rupture is a recognized complication of iliac angioplasty and stenting. Rupture of the external iliac artery is more common than that of the common iliac artery. Although rare, when it does occur, life-threatening hemorrhage can occur within a very short space of time. Thus, knowledge of how to manage this complication and the steps involved should be something all interventional radiologists involved in iliac intervention should be familiar with. Stent grafts of an appropriate size should always be available before commencing such procedures. The role of each team member should also be clarified before the procedure should the patient become hemodynamically compromised.

The two most important aspects of management are to instigate temporizing measures to stop the bleeding from the ruptured artery (i.e., reinflate the angioplasty balloon or, failing this, place an occlusion balloon) and to resuscitate the patient. Once the immediate emergency situation has been stabilized, thought can then be turned to definitive management of the rupture with a stent graft. This will usually require bilateral femoral access, one access site to control bleeding (usually the contralateral) and the other to deploy the stent graft in order to minimize further blood loss. The choice of balloon expandable or self-expanding stent graft will be dictated by the device stocked by individual departments. Either is suitable in this situation, as long as a device of appropriate diameter and length is available. It is often prudent to ask a colleague for help, if available, as it is simpler and quicker to manage sequential occlusion balloon deflation and stent graft placement with two pairs of hands!

Tips

- Arterial rupture is a rare, but potentially catastrophic complication of vascular intervention.
- The external iliac artery is particularly prone to this complication.
- Before embarking on intervention in the iliac artery ensure an appropriate stent graft is available to treat a rupture.
- Recognition of iliac artery rupture and prompt action to stop bleeding are paramount to prevent rapid demise of the patient.
- As with any life-threatening complication, the most important steps are to temporize the immediate situation and resuscitate the patient.

- Reinflation of the angioplasty balloon across the rupture site will stem any hemorrhage to give time for resuscitation and instigate definitive treatment.
- An additional access site and an extra pair of hands (ask a friendly colleague!) are extremely useful to allow simultaneous control of bleeding and placement of stent grafts.

Commentary

Most vascular interventional radiologists will experience this complication at some point in their career. The approach described here is the treatment option of choice. Although it occurs rarely, it is important to act promptly to minimize hemorrhage. In this case the authors were able to access the ipsilateral femoral artery and get past the inflated angioplasty balloon quite promptly, but this is not always easy to do, especially when under pressure. In these situations, bilateral femoral access from the outset has merits with retrograde ipsilateral stenting over a snared wire even when recanalization has occurred from the contralateral approach. Having dual access already in place makes deployment of a covered stent much faster and easier.

It is recommended that iliac angioplasty should not be performed unless a stent graft is available. However, there are other alternatives to the management of this complication. The iliac artery could be embolized in the acute situation, and the patient later referred for bypass surgery if necessary. Or emergency bypass surgery can be performed, in which case the balloon catheter will be left inflated while the patient is transferred to surgery.

Further Reading

Allaire E, Melliere D, Poussier B, Kobeiter H, Desgranges P, Becquemin JP. Iliac artery rupture during balloon dilatation: what treatment? Ann Vasc Surg. 2003;17(3):306–14.

Chatziioannou A, Mourikis D, Katsimilis J, Skiadas V, Koutoulidis V, Katsenis K, Vlahos L. Acute iliac artery rupture: endovascular treatment. Cardiovasc Intervent Radiol. 2007;30(2):281–5.

Chapter 13
Detachment of a Balloon-Expandable Stent from the Balloon and the Wire

Robert P. Allison, Anna Maria Belli, Joo-Young Chun, Raymond Chung, Raj Das, Andrew England, Karen Flood, Marie-France Giroux, Richard G. McWilliams, Robert Morgan, Nik Papadakos, Jai V. Patel, Raf Patel, Uday Patel, Lakshmi Ratnam, Reddi Prasad Yadavali, and John Rose

Abstract This case illustrates how a detached stent can be safely fixed and deployed in a suitable vessel. Other methods for stent retrieval are also reviewed.

Keywords Complications • Stenting • Stent detachment • Snare

R.P. Allison
Department of Interventional Radiology, University Hospitals Southampton, Southampton, Hampshire, UK

A.M. Belli
Department of Radiology, St. George's Hospital and Medical School, Blackshaw Road, London SW17 0RE, UK
e-mail: anna.belli@stgeorges.nhs.uk

J.-Y. Chun • R. Chung • R. Das
R. Morgan • N. Papadakos
Department of Radiology, St. George's Hospital, London, UK

A. England
Department of Radiography, University of Salford, Manchester, UK

K. Flood
Department of Vascular Radiology, Leeds General Infirmary,
Leeds, UK

M.-F. Giroux
Department of Radiology, CHUM-Centre Hospitalier
de l'Université de Montréal, Montreal, QC, Canada

R.G. McWilliams
Department of Radiology, Royal Liverpool University Hospital,
Liverpool, UK

J.V. Patel
Department of Radiology, The Leeds Teaching Hospitals NHS Trust,
Leeds, West Yorkshire, UK

R. Patel
Department of Radiology,
The Leeds Teaching Hospitals NHS Trust,
Leeds, West Yorkshire, UK
e-mail: rafpatel@gmail.com

U. Patel
Department of Diagnostic Radiology, St. George's Hospital and
Medical School, Blackshaw Road, SW17 0QT London, UK
e-mail: uday.patel@stgeorges.nhs.uk

L. Ratnam
Department of Radiology, St. George's Hospital, Blackshaw Road,
SW17 0QT London, UK
e-mail: lakshmi.ratnam@nhs.net

R.P. Yadavali
Department of Radiology, Aberdeen Royal Infirmary, Aberdeen, UK

J. Rose
Department of Interventional Radiology, Freeman Hospital,
Newcastle Upon Tyne Hospitals NHS Trust, Newcastle upon Tyne, UK

Case History

A 68-year-old male presented with a history of a left ankle ulcer and short-distance bilateral disabling claudication. Magnetic resonance angiography (MRA) demonstrated bilateral significant common iliac stenoses with an occlusion of the left external iliac, common femoral and superficial femoral arteries. Bilateral iliac angioplasty and stenting from a right femoral retrograde approach was planned prior to a surgical left femoropopliteal bypass graft.

Procedure

A 6-Fr retrograde right CFA puncture was performed. Angioplasty was unsuccessful as the right common iliac and external iliac stenoses were heavily calcified and were therefore stented. Next, the left EIA occlusion was traversed with a guidewire advanced into a patent profunda femoris artery. However, a long 6-Fr access sheath would not track across the angled aortic bifurcation.

An attempt was made to advance a 9 mm × 6 cm balloon-expandable stent contralaterally from the right femoral access site to stent the left EIA occlusion. However, there was resistance on advancing the stent. This resulted in inadvertent fracture of the right femoral arterial access sheath at the hub, withdrawal of the wire, and detachment of the stent from the delivery catheter. The unexpanded stent at this stage lay free within the right iliac artery (Fig. 13.1a).

The damaged right femoral access sheath was removed after reintroduction of the guidewire and exchanged for a new 6-Fr sheath. The mobile unexpanded stent in the right external iliac artery was fixed in place by deploying a new 9 mm × 6 cm balloon-expandable stent within it (Fig. 13.1b, c). The left iliac occlusion (Fig. 13.2a) was traversed again and stented with self-expanding stents (Fig. 13.2b).

The patient's symptoms improved significantly post-procedure, and there have been no adverse sequelae from the additional stents in the right external iliac artery.

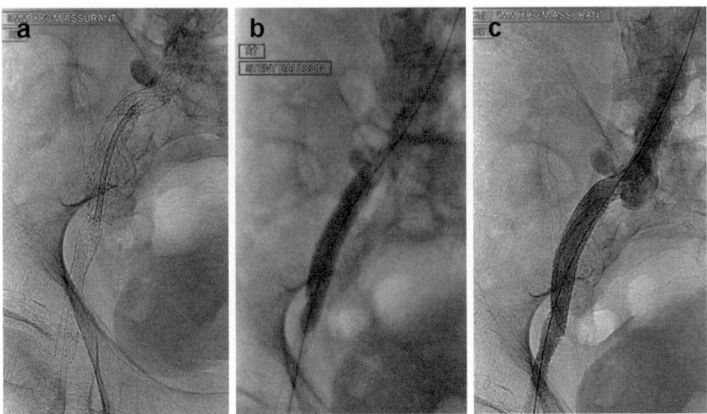

Figure 13.1 (a) Detached balloon-mounted stent lying free within already stented right CIA/EIA; (b) the detached stent is fixed in place by positioning another balloon-expandable stent across it; (c) check angiogram after fixing the detached balloon in place demonstrates satisfactory flow

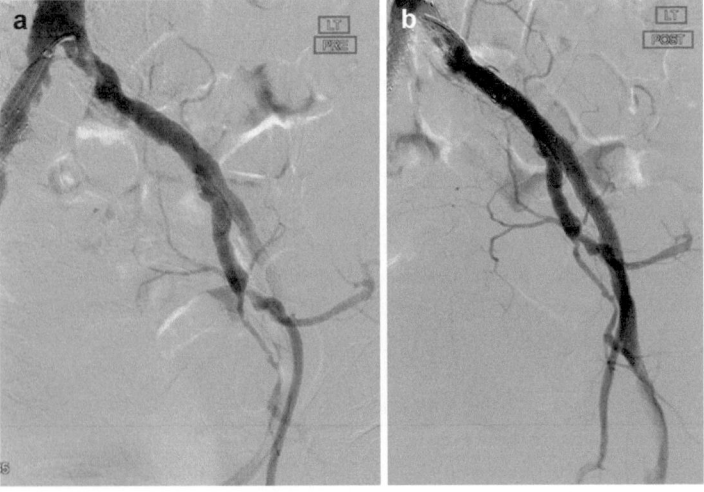

Figure 13.2 (a) Digital subtraction angiogram demonstrates a left EIA occlusion; (b) post-procedure angiogram demonstrating a patent left iliac arterial system after stenting with self-expandable stents in the left CIA and EIA

Discussion

Detachment of a stent is a potentially disastrous complication, which is more likely to occur when advancing stents through heavily calcified stenoses or around sharp angulations. To overcome this, tight stenoses can be pre-dilated. A guide catheter or sheath can also be used to navigate beyond the target lesion and deliver the stent, following which the stent can be "unsheathed" by withdrawing the guide catheter or sheath prior to deploying the stent at the desired location.

A number of options are available for the management of a detached balloon-mounted stent. If noticed early and the stent remains on the balloon but has moved in relation to the balloon markers, then any movement or deployment of the balloon should be attempted in a very controlled manner as asymmetrical balloon inflation may detach the stent to an undesirable location. If the stent remains on the balloon but has begun to move off the balloon, then partial balloon inflation may help grip the stent and allow it to be repositioned. If this is unsuccessful, attempts may be made to retrieve the stent, or conversely it may be less harmful to deploy the stent in an alternative suitably sized vessel.

If a balloon-expandable stent detaches from the balloon but remains on the catheter shaft, it may be removed by withdrawing the catheter shaft into the groin sheath. The sheath can then be removed with the stent in situ and exchanged while retaining wire access.

If a balloon-mounted stent detaches off the balloon and the catheter but remains on the wire, then it may be possible to recapture the stent by passing a low profile balloon along the wire to grip the stent. Alternatively, a snare device can be used. The snare can be passed over the wire from the same access site to capture and retrieve the stent into the sheath for removal. If this is unsuccessful, then a snare can be inserted from another access site to capture the distal end of the wire, on which the stent is, to establish a through-and-through wire position from which the stent cannot be "lost" and can be retrieved with a snare.

Detachment of a balloon-mounted stent off the wire, as in this case, can be more problematic. If the stent is in a suitable location such as an iliac artery, it may be simpler to crush and fix the stent in place with another stent. If the stent is in an unsuitable location then retrieval with a snare can be attempted.

This case illustrates how a detached stent can be safely fixed and deployed in a suitable vessel. This technique is usually significantly easier, carries less risks of vascular access complications or dissection, and requires less time then retrieving the detached stent.

Tips

- Try to anticipate potential detachment of a balloon-mounted stent especially when negotiating tight stenoses or acute angles.
- A detached stent can be managed in a variety of ways dependent on whether it remains on the wire, on the catheter shaft or free in the vessel.
- A detached stent can be fixed safely in an alternative vessel by another stent to prevent any future stent migration or embolization.

Commentary

Factors which increase the likelihood of dislodging a stent include heavy calcification, tortuosity, and a severe stenosis or occlusion. The authors comprehensively describe various methods used to secure a dislodged balloon-mounted stent. An alternative approach is to secure ipsilateral access for iliac angioplasty and stenting even if the occlusion or stenosis can only be crossed from a contralateral approach initially (then snare the wire via an ipsilateral access). Even though this requires dual groin punctures, in cases such as this, the risk of detachment of a stent is significantly reduced and more importantly; should there be an arterial rupture, you are much better placed to treat this (see previous case of iatrogenic iliac artery rupture, Chap. 12).

Further Reading

Feldman T. Retrieval techniques for dislodged stents. Catheter Cardiovasc Interv. 1999;47:325–6.

Meisel SR, DiLeo J, Rajakaruna M, Pace B, Frankel R, Shani J. A technique to retrieve stents dislodged in the coronary artery followed by fixation in the iliac artery by means of balloon angioplasty and peripheral stent deployment. Catheter Cardiovasc Interv. 2000; 49(1):77–81.

Chapter 14
Migration of Common Hepatic Artery Stent Graft Occluding Right Hepatic Artery Flow

Robert P. Allison, Anna Maria Belli, Joo-Young Chun, Raymond Chung, Raj Das, Andrew England, Karen Flood, Marie-France Giroux, Richard G. McWilliams, Robert Morgan, Nik Papadakos, Jai V. Patel, Raf Patel, Uday Patel, Lakshmi Ratnam, Reddi Prasad Yadavali, and John Rose

Abstract This case illustrates the technique of using adjacent/buttress stenting to keep open an artery compromised by a maldeployed stent graft.

Keywords Complication • Stenting • Stent malposition

R.P. Allison
Department of Interventional Radiology,
University Hospitals Southampton,
Southampton, Hampshire, UK

A.M. Belli
Department of Radiology,
St. George's Hospital and Medical School,
Blackshaw Road, London SW17 0RE, UK
e-mail: anna.belli@stgeorges.nhs.uk

J.-Y. Chun • R. Chung • R. Das
R. Morgan • N. Papadakos
Department of Radiology, St. George's Hospital, London, UK

A. England
Department of Radiography, University of Salford, Manchester, UK

K. Flood
Department of Vascular Radiology,
Leeds General Infirmary, Leeds, UK

M.-F. Giroux
Department of Radiology,
CHUM-Centre Hospitalier de l'Université de Montréal,
Montreal, QC, Canada

R.G. McWilliams
Department of Radiology,
Royal Liverpool University Hospital, Liverpool, UK

J.V. Patel
Department of Radiology,
The Leeds Teaching Hospitals NHS Trust,
Leeds, West Yorkshire, UK

R. Patel
Department of Radiology,
The Leeds Teaching Hospitals NHS Trust,
Leeds, West Yorkshire, UK
e-mail: rafpatel@gmail.com

U. Patel
Department of Diagnostic Radiology,
St. George's Hospital and Medical School,
Blackshaw Road, SW17 0QT London, UK
e-mail: uday.patel@stgeorges.nhs.uk

L. Ratnam
Department of Radiology,
St. George's Hospital,
Blackshaw Road, SW17 0QT London, UK
e-mail: lakshmi.ratnam@nhs.net

R.P. Yadavali
Department of Radiology,
Aberdeen Royal Infirmary, Aberdeen, UK

J. Rose
Department of Interventional Radiology,
Freeman Hospital, Newcastle Upon Tyne Hospitals NHS Trust,
Newcastle upon Tyne, UK

Chapter 14. Migration of Common Hepatic Artery Stent

Case History

A 65-year-old lady was transferred to our hospital post Whipple procedure for removal of a pancreatic head tumor. Following this she had episodes of recurrent upper GI bleeding requiring multiple blood transfusions. CT and catheter angiography at another institution had not shown a definite source of the bleed. Gastroduodenal artery (GDA) stump coil embolization had been performed previously. Bleeding was ongoing, and after clinical discussion, it was decided that further mesenteric angiography with stent-graft placement in the hepatic artery, across the GDA stump would be carried out, to isolate the GDA.

Procedure

Initial angiography was performed via a right retrograde common femoral arterial puncture and catheterization of the coeliac and superior mesenteric arteries with a Simmons 2 catheter. No active bleed or false aneurysm from the coeliac or hepatic arteries was seen, and the GDA stump could be visualized. Catheter position in the coeliac axis was unstable, and despite exchanging for Cobra and Berenstein catheters, it was difficult to achieve a stable position across the GDA. This was finally achieved using a 7-Fr-long sheath via a left brachial artery approach (Fig. 14.1).

A 7×22 mm balloon-expandable stent graft was passed along the coeliac artery and across the GDA stump, but this was difficult to track distally. Angiography confirmed a suitable pre-deployment position, but after deployment it was noted that the distal end of the stent graft had deployed into the left hepatic artery (HA), covering the origin of the right HA (Fig. 14.2a). The right HA was catheterized using a coaxial microcatheter, which was exchanged for a platinum plus wire. A 5×18 mm balloon-expandable stent was used as a buttressing stent in the right HA, placed parallel and adjacent to the stent graft (Fig. 14.2b). Completion angiography

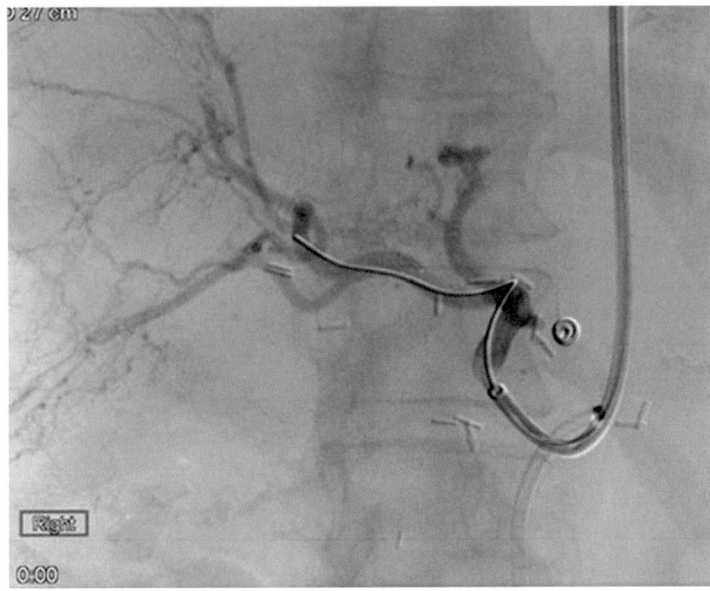

Figure 14.1 Angiography performed via 7-Fr-long sheath in coeliac axis, via left brachial artery approach. No contrast extravasation or false aneurysm identified

demonstrated restored flow within the RHA and satisfactory stent-graft placement. Clinical re-bleeding has not occurred post procedure.

Discussion

Endovascular treatment is the favored management of hemorrhage following pancreaticoduodenectomy. The source of ongoing intermittent hemorrhage can often be difficult to confirm on CT or catheter angiography. In this case, although no contrast extravasation or pseudoaneurysm had been identified, the GDA was the presumed source of bleeding and was excluded from the circulation using a stent graft in the common hepatic artery, across the GDA origin.

Chapter 14. Migration of Common Hepatic Artery Stent

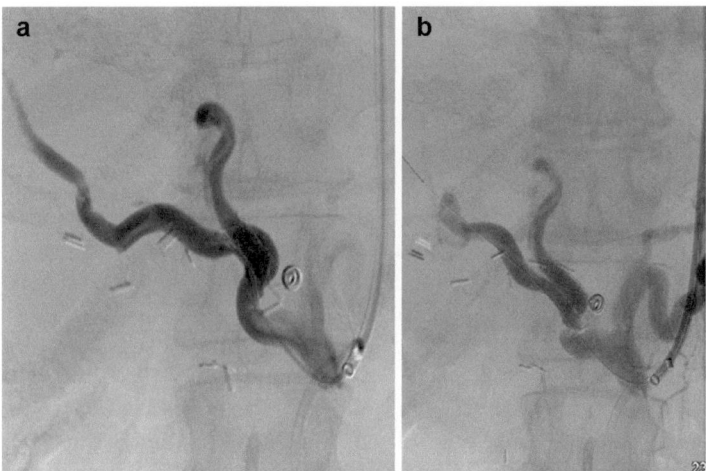

FIGURE 14.2 (**a**) Proximal end of stent graft deployed in left HA crossing the origin of right HA; (**b**) completion hepatic angiography demonstrating good left and right HA flow following RHA buttressing stent

Initially access from the femoral artery did not provide a stable enough catheter position in the coeliac access to allow a wire to cross the GDA origin from the common hepatic artery. A 7-F-long sheath from the left brachial approach improved stability; however, there were still difficulties maintaining position. The microcatheter wire and catheter were able to pass into the left/right hepatic arteries, but it was difficult to track a stiffer, i.e., platinum plus, wire across for deployment of the stent graft. Tracking of the stent graft was difficult and required a large amount of forward pressure to encourage forward movement. The position appeared satisfactory before deployment, but malpositioning was seen on the post-deployment angiogram. The stent graft had slipped forward and the right hepatic arterial flow was compromised. There was a high risk of ischemic compromise to the liver if left untreated. A parallel buttressing stent was placed to allow blood flow into the right hepatic artery.

Tips

- CT angiography (CTA) is the most sensitive investigation for demonstrating active hemorrhage and should be the first-line investigation in the majority of postoperative patients.
- In a patient with continuing postoperative hemorrhage requiring blood transfusions, potential sites for bleeding should be treated even though active bleeding may not be visualized on angiography.
- Consider arm arterial access for difficult catheterization of the mesenteric arteries.
- Once deployed, stent grafts cannot be easily repositioned.
- If there is no arterial compromise, further stent-graft deployment can be used to extend/ensure coverage of the required area.
- If there is compromised blood flow to an artery, consider adjacent or buttressing stenting.
- Surgical removal of the stent graft could be considered if other methods are unsuccessful.

Commentary

Coil embolization or occlusion of the hepatic artery does not usually compromise liver function due to the dual blood supply to the liver from the hepatic artery and the portal vein. The exceptions to this are in cases where the portal vein is occluded, in liver transplant patients and in some postoperative situations where embolization of the hepatic artery has an adverse consequence to distal perfusion. Patency of the portal vein is confirmed by performing a prolonged selective celiac artery run; filling of the portal vein is seen after filling of the celiac axis.

Stent grafts are a suitable alternative in allowing treatment of hemorrhage while maintaining arterial perfusion. Balloon-mounted stent grafts allow more precise placement and have a greater radial strength compared to non-balloon-mounted stent grafts.

Where a stent graft has been maldeployed, several strategies are available. The first is to assess if there is any compromise from the malposition. If there is no consequence from leaving the stent where it is, this is often the best course. The authors have demonstrated effectively the technique of using an additional stent to keep open the compromised artery.

If a stent is not fully expanded, inflating an angioplasty balloon within the stent graft may allow it to be moved into a more appropriate position; this must be done with caution to avoid damaging the vessel or causing a perforation.

Further Reading

Makowiec F, Riediger H, Euringer W, Uhl M, Hopt UT, Adam U. Management of delayed visceral arterial bleeding after pancreatic head resection. J Gastrointest Surg. 2005;9(9):1293–9.

Rami P, Williams D, Forauer A, Cwikiel W. Stent-graft treatment of patients with acute bleeding from hepatic artery branches. Cardiovasc Intervent Radiol. 2005;28:153–8.

Yekebas EF, Wolfram L, Cataldegirmen G, et al. Postpancreatectomy hemorrhage: diagnosis and treatment: an analysis in 1669 consecutive pancreatic resections. Ann Surg. 2007;246(2):269–80.

Chapter 15
Migrated Stent Graft During TIPS Revision

Robert P. Allison, Anna Maria Belli, Joo-Young Chun, Raymond Chung, Raj Das, Andrew England, Karen Flood, Marie-France Giroux, Richard G. McWilliams, Robert Morgan, Nik Papadakos, Jai V. Patel, Raf Patel, Uday Patel, Lakshmi Ratnam, Reddi Prasad Yadavali, and John Rose

Abstract This case demonstrates how to capture and redeploy a migrated stent graft. Principles of safe repositioning are discussed.

Keywords Complications • Migrated stent graft • Snare

R.P. Allison
Department of Interventional Radiology, University Hospitals Southampton, Southampton, Hampshire, UK

A.M. Belli
Department of Radiology, St. George's Hospital and Medical School, Blackshaw Road, London SW17 0RE, UK
e-mail: anna.belli@stgeorges.nhs.uk

J.-Y. Chun • R. Chung • R. Das
R. Morgan • N. Papadakos
Department of Radiology, St. George's Hospital, London, UK

A. England
Department of Radiography, University of Salford,
Manchester, UK

K. Flood
Department of Vascular Radiology, Leeds General Infirmary,
Leeds, UK

M.-F. Giroux
Department of Radiology, CHUM-Centre Hospitalier de
l'Université de Montréal, Montreal, QC, Canada

R.G. McWilliams
Department of Radiology, Royal Liverpool University Hospital,
Liverpool, UK

J.V. Patel
Department of Radiology, The Leeds Teaching Hospitals NHS Trust,
Leeds, West Yorkshire, UK

R. Patel
Department of Radiology,
The Leeds Teaching Hospitals NHS Trust,
Leeds, West Yorkshire, UK
e-mail: rafpatel@gmail.com

U. Patel
Department of Diagnostic Radiology, St. George's Hospital and
Medical School, Blackshaw Road, SW17 0QT London, UK
e-mail: uday.patel@stgeorges.nhs.uk

L. Ratnam
Department of Radiology, St. George's Hospital, Blackshaw Road,
SW17 0QT London, UK
e-mail: lakshmi.ratnam@nhs.net

R.P. Yadavali
Department of Radiology, Aberdeen Royal Infirmary, Aberdeen, UK

J. Rose
Department of Interventional Radiology, Freeman Hospital,
Newcastle Upon Tyne Hospitals NHS Trust, Newcastle upon Tyne, UK

Case History

A 49-year-old man with cirrhosis secondary to hepatitis C underwent a transjugular intrahepatic portosystemic shunt (TIPS) procedure for drug-resistant ascites. The TIPS was fashioned between the right portal vein and right hepatic vein using a self-expanding bare-metal stent. On day 12 a routine TIPS Doppler ultrasound scan revealed a significant velocity gradient at the portal venous end of the TIPS consistent with a stenosis. A TIPS venogram was performed with a view to placing a stent graft through the TIPS track.

Procedure

A balloon-expandable stent graft (9–12 mm) was placed onto a balloon and deployed within the TIPS via the right internal jugular vein. During balloon inflation, the stent graft was noted to migrate along the angioplasty balloon due to the balloon inflating from its distal extent. The stent graft failed to engage within the TIPS and migrated along the wire, into the superior vena cava (SVC) (Fig. 15.1a). Despite repeated attempts, the stent graft would not pass back into the TIPS. Further venography showed the right brachiocephalic vein to be of an appropriate size (15 mm) to deploy the stent graft. In order to prevent loss of the stent graft into the right atrium, through-and-through access was achieved by passing a second wire down the right jugular sheath, through the stent graft and snaring it from a second sheath placed in the right femoral vein (Fig. 15.1b, c). A 15 mm angioplasty balloon was then passed down this wire and partially inflated within the stent graft (Fig. 15.2a). The balloon was withdrawn with the stent graft into the right brachiocephalic vein and fully inflated. Following what seemed to be a deployed good position, the stent graft was seen to migrate back into the SVC once the balloon was deflated. The same maneuver was repeated, this time using a 20 mm balloon (Fig. 15.2b). Despite an apparent initially successful deployment, the stent graft again migrated

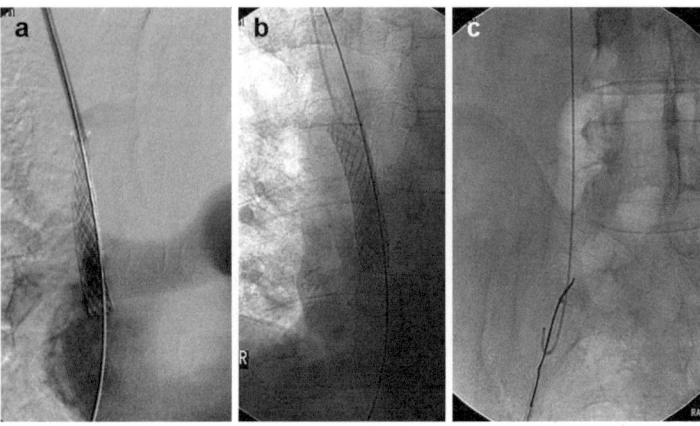

FIGURE 15.1 (**a**) Migrated stent graft lying within the superior vena cava (*SVC*); (**b**) catheter passed through the stent graft; and (**c**) a wire snared from the femoral vein to provide through-and-through access and to prevent inadvertent "loss" of the stent graft into the right atrium

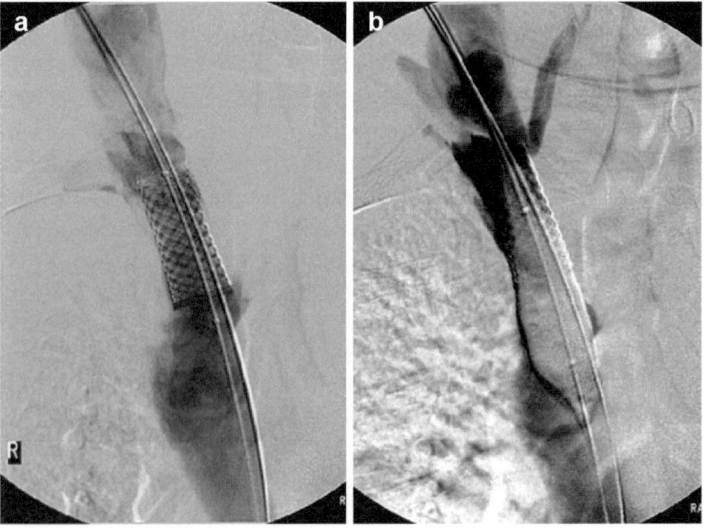

FIGURE 15.2 (**a**) Stent graft inflated to 15 mm within the right brachiocephalic vein; (**b**) same maneuver repeated with a 20 mm balloon

Chapter 15. Migrated Stent Graft During TIPS Revision 109

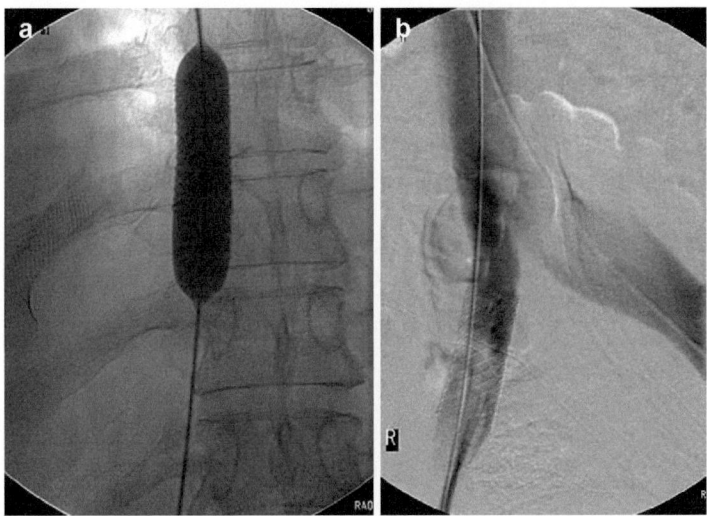

FIGURE 15.3 (**a**) 20 mm balloon inflated within the stent graft and negotiated into the SVC; (**b**) final position within the right common iliac vein, anchored in place with a 20 mm self-expanding metal stent

back into the SVC, and it was apparent that the stent graft would not remain in a stable position within the brachiocephalic vein. The 20 mm balloon was partially reinflated within the stent graft and the combination gently passed down into the IVC and eventually into the right common iliac vein (CIV) (Fig. 15.3a). Once there, the balloon was fully inflated and the stent graft now appeared to be in a stable position. A 20 mm self-expanding bare-metal stent was placed to ensure anchorage of the stent graft within the CIV (Fig. 15.3b).

Discussion

Stent migration can occur during their placement in either the arterial or venous system. This can occur due to inadequate sizing with either self-expanding or balloon-expandable stents and is more likely in the venous system during movement of balloon-expandable stents while advancing them to the target site or during balloon inflation. Self-expanding stents can move forward during deployment. There are a number of options available for retrieving or "salvaging" a migrated stent. One option is to collapse the proximal end of the stent with a snare to prevent it from "catching" on the vessel wall and then pull it out through the access sheath. This can be a good option for a self-expanding stent as the remainder of the stent will collapse as it is pulled through the sheath (i.e., the reverse action to stent deployment). It is more problematic with balloon-expandable stent, where the whole of the stent needs to be crushed down with the snare before it can be retrieved. If a stent migrates into a precarious position, e.g., the heart, consider achieving through-and-through wire access, as this way there is no chance of the stent coming off the wire, making a bad situation worse! If retrieval is not possible, the next option would be to place the stent in a "safe" position at an alternative site. With bare-metal stents this may involve placing the stent across a branch vessel. In general, a large branch vessel will remain patent, e.g., the internal iliac artery when stents are placed from the common iliac into the external iliac artery. However, stent grafts require more careful consideration as any side branches that are covered will, by necessity, occlude. If all else fails, the stent may have to be "moved" to a superficial vessel and then retrieved via a surgical cutdown.

This case study is somewhat historical in that TIPS procedures are now often performed placing dedicated TIPS stent grafts during the primary intervention. Re-interventions in a bare-metal TIPS would also involve such self-expanding stent grafts. However, it does illustrate some of the strategies that can be employed when faced with a migrated stent or stent graft in any situation.

Tips

- Migration of stents can occur during vascular interventions.
- There is more potential for venous stents to migrate to "unfavorable" anatomical sites.

Chapter 15. Migrated Stent Graft During TIPS Revision 111

- A migrated stent that remains on a guide wire is more readily salvaged than one that lies free in the vessel.
- Consider a through-and-through wire to prevent loss of the stent off the wire.
- A number of options can be considered to salvage a migrated stent:
  1. Snare and retrieve.
  2. Redeploy in an alternative vessel.
  3. Snare and surgically remove.
- In the case of stent grafts, carefully consider the consequences of any branch vessel coverage.

Commentary

Stent migration is a particular problem in venous interventions. Even seemingly tight stenoses can expand easily, leading to inadequate sizing and migration. Hand-crimped balloon-expandable stents can be relatively easily dislodged either during passage through a tight stenosis or during balloon inflation, as in the case described here. This case demonstrates the thought processes and actions to retrieve a complication, especially when the first option of deployment in the brachiocephalic vein failed and the stent had to be negotiated down to the common iliac vein. If a stent seems unstable in its position in a vein, even if it is in a currently acceptable location, movement is likely to occur and in such situations anchoring the stent with a larger diameter stent will prevent movement.

Further Reading

Bagul NB, Moth P, Menon NJ, Myint F, Hamilton G. Migration of superior vena cava stent. J Cardiothorac Surg. 2008;3:12.

Feldman T. Retrieval techniques for dislodged stents. Catheter Cardiovasc Interv. 1999;47:325–6.

Rossle M, Gerbes AL. TIPS for the treatment of refractory ascites, hepatorenal syndrome and hepatic hydrothorax: a critical update. Gut. 2010;59(7):988–1000.

Taylor JD, Lehmann ED, Belli A-M, Nicholson AA, Kessel D, Robertson IR, Pollock G, Morgan RA. Strategies for the management of SVC stent migration into the right atrium. Cardiovasc Intervent Radiol. 2007;30:1003–9.

Yang Z, Han G, Wu Q, Ye X, Jin Z, Yin Z, Qi X, Bai M, Wu K, Fan D. Patency and clinical outcomes of transjugular intrahepatic portosystemic shunt with polytetrafluoroethylene-covered stents versus bare stents: a meta-analysis. J Gastroenterol Hepatol. 2010;25(11):1718–25.

Chapter 16
Type 1A Endoleak Following EVAR Treated with a Proximal Cuff

Robert P. Allison, Anna Maria Belli, Joo-Young Chun, Raymond Chung, Raj Das, Andrew England, Karen Flood, Marie-France Giroux, Richard G. McWilliams, Robert Morgan, Nik Papadakos, Jai V. Patel, Raf Patel, Uday Patel, Lakshmi Ratnam, Reddi Prasad Yadavali, and John Rose

Abstract This case illustrates management of a proximal type 1 endoleak post EVAR with a proximal cuff. Management of the resulting compromise to a renal artery is also illustrated.

Keywords Complications • EVAR • Type 1 endoleak • Proximal cuff

---

R.P. Allison
Department of Interventional Radiology,
University Hospitals Southampton,
Southampton, Hampshire, UK

A.M. Belli
Department of Radiology,
St. George's Hospital and Medical School,
Blackshaw Road, London SW17 0RE, UK
e-mail: anna.belli@stgeorges.nhs.uk

J.-Y. Chun • R. Chung • R. Das
R. Morgan • N. Papadakos
Department of Radiology,
St. George's Hospital, London, UK

A. England
Department of Radiography,
University of Salford, Manchester, UK

K. Flood
Department of Vascular Radiology,
Leeds General Infirmary, Leeds, UK

M.-F. Giroux
Department of Radiology,
CHUM-Centre Hospitalier de l'Université de Montréal,
Montreal, QC, Canada

R.G. McWilliams
Department of Radiology, Royal Liverpool University Hospital,
Liverpool, UK

J.V. Patel
Department of Radiology,
The Leeds Teaching Hospitals NHS Trust,
Leeds, West Yorkshire, UK

R. Patel
Department of Radiology,
The Leeds Teaching Hospitals NHS Trust,
Leeds, West Yorkshire, UK
e-mail: rafpatel@gmail.com

U. Patel
Department of Diagnostic Radiology,
St. George's Hospital and Medical School,
Blackshaw Road, SW17 0QT London, UK
e-mail: uday.patel@stgeorges.nhs.uk

L. Ratnam
Department of Radiology,
St. George's Hospital, Blackshaw Road, SW17 0QT London, UK
e-mail: lakshmi.ratnam@nhs.net

R.P. Yadavali
Department of Radiology,
Aberdeen Royal Infirmary, Aberdeen, UK

J. Rose
Department of Interventional Radiology,
Freeman Hospital, Newcastle Upon Tyne Hospitals NHS Trust,
Newcastle upon Tyne, UK

Case History

A 67-year-old man with an asymptomatic 7.3 cm AAA was referred for EVAR, and an Endurant bifurcated device (Medtronic Santa Rosa, CA) was implanted. Completion angiography confirmed successful deployment of the stent graft and the absence of any graft-related endoleak. The fabric markers were a few millimeters below the inferior margin of the renal arteries, but there appeared to be adequate apposition of fabric in the neck.

At 1-month follow-up CT scan, there was no evidence of a proximal type 1 endoleak (Fig. 16.1a), but a type 2 endoleak could be seen and appeared to be communicating with the 3rd and 4th lumbar arteries and IMA. At the 1-year CT scan, there was persistence of the previously identified type 2 endoleak, and there was a new proximal type 1 endoleak (Fig. 16.1b). In addition the aneurysm had increased in diameter to 8.1 cm. The patient underwent urgent catheter angiography to confirm the etiology of the endoleak and provide a definitive treatment plan. Aortography, with angulation of the image intensifier to correct for aortic neck tortuosity, revealed 7 mm of uncovered aortic neck between the lowest renal artery (right) and the proximal device fabric markers. Both the proximal type 1 (Fig. 16.2a) and the distal type 2 endoleaks were confirmed.

Procedure

The following day the patient was taken back to theater. A proximal cuff was implanted and molded using a Coda balloon (Cook INC, Bloomington, IN) (Fig. 16.2b, c). Subsequent angiography suggested that there may be some minor fabric encroachment to the left renal artery (Fig. 16.3a). Fluoroscopic images also raised the possibility that a stent-graft anchoring barb may be projecting into the left renal artery ostium. This could make renal artery access difficult and could act as a snagging point for any endovascular devices. Despite this, the fabric

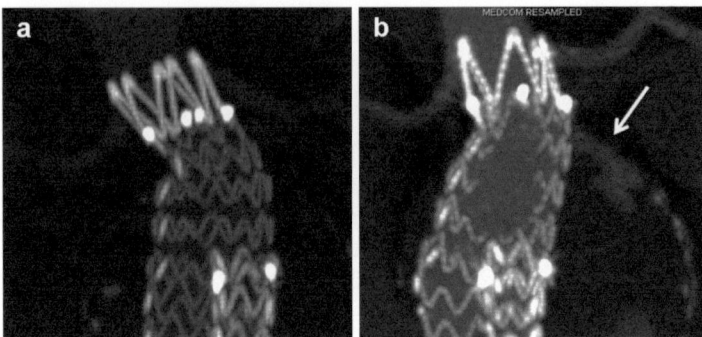

FIGURE 16.1 (**a**) First postoperative CT scan (1-month). Coronal reformatted MIP image demonstrating the deployment position. The fabric markers are below the renal arteries and there is no type 1 proximal endoleak; (**b**) 1-year follow-up CT scan. Coronal reformatted MIP image demonstrating a proximal type 1 endoleak (*arrow*), the renal fabric markers are in the mid-aortic neck

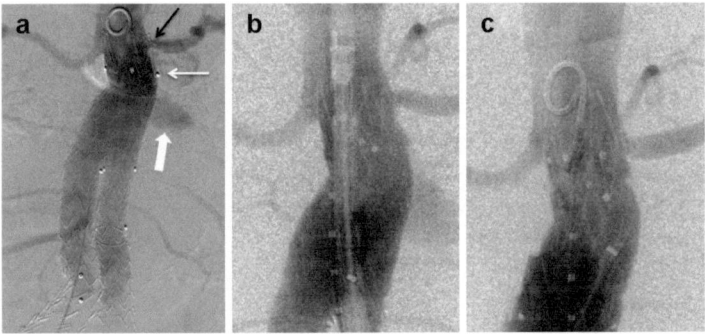

FIGURE 16.2 (**a**) Follow-up catheter aortogram demonstrating a proximal type 1 endoleak (*block white arrow*). Note the position of the fabric markers in the mid-aortic neck (*white arrow*) and the barb projecting into the origin of the left renal artery (*black arrow*); (**b**) fluoroscopy image immediately before the deployment of the proximal aortic cuff; (**c**) angiogram following deployment of the proximal cuff and molding with a Coda balloon. The proximal type 1 endoleak is now absent, and there is now fabric covering the whole of the infrarenal aortic neck

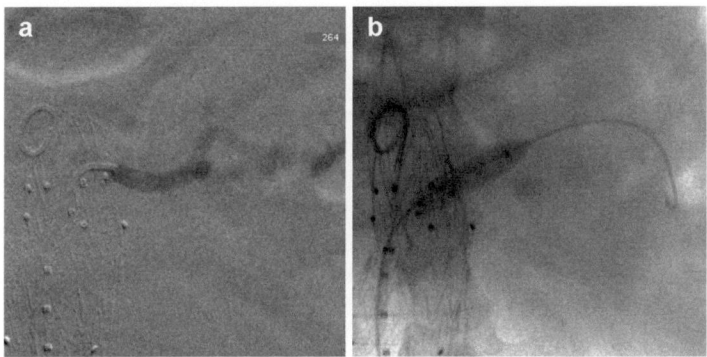

Figure 16.3 (**a**) There was some suspicion that the fabric on the proximal cuff was impinging on the blood flow into the left renal artery. A selective renal angiogram confirmed that the fabric marker (sitting slightly lower than the top of the fabric) was sitting on the inferior margin of the left renal artery ostium; (**b**) a balloon-expandable stent was deployed into the origin of the left renal artery. On completion angiography there was good flow into both renal arteries and there was no proximal type 1 endoleak

encroachment was treated by implantation of a Palmaz Genesis (Cordis, Miami, FL) balloon-expandable stent (Fig. 16.3b). Completion angiography showed resolution of the proximal type 1 endoleak and good flow into both renal arteries. The patient recovered from surgery and was discharged home.

Discussion

Proximal type 1 endoleaks are caused by a failure to achieve a circumferential seal at the proximal attachment site. Early (<30-days) proximal type 1 endoleaks are generally seen on intraoperative imaging and occur in 5–10 % of all EVAR procedures. Late (>30-days) endoleaks are usually associated with a secondary complication such as device migration, persistent type 2 endoleaks or aortic neck enlargement. Urgent treatment is required for all proximal endoleaks since they have been associated with an increased risk of aneurysm rupture.

Early proximal type 1 endoleaks may be treated with a Palmaz stent (Cordis, Miami, FL) or aortic cuff if they fail to respond to initial balloon molding. Late leaks respond less well to simple balloon molding and require a more definitive solution. A proximal aortic cuff is only an option for patients where there is a section of the aortic neck which has been left uncovered, for these patients either the stent graft has been deployed low or the device has migrated distally. The insertion of a proximal cuff can be difficult and is not without risks. Deploying the cuff too high may compromise the renal blood supply, whereas a low deployment may allow persistence of the endoleak. Reports in the literature suggest that technical success is achieved in only around 50 % of cases. In our case there was full resolution of the endoleak but with impingement on the origin of the left renal artery.

A Palmaz stent is used in patients where there is good fabric coverage of the aortic neck. In these cases there may be a sizing problem, which has allowed antegrade blood flow into the aneurysm sac or severe aortic neck angulation, tortuosity, or mural thrombus which has resulted in incomplete apposition of the device and the resultant endoleak. Dilatation of the aortic neck during follow-up may also lead to a loss of seal and is a further risk factor for a proximal type 1 endoleak.

Patients with short, wide, or thrombus-lined aortic necks may not be suitable for one of the above treatment options. Conversion to open repair or surgical banding of the aortic neck is a possibility but is more invasive and is associated with high mortality and morbidity. Many patients that are referred for EVAR have existing medical comorbidities that place them at high risk for open aneurysm surgery. A more complex and more expensive endovascular solution is implantation of a fenestrated cuff. This requires careful planning and manufacturing time but is an option in the presence of challenging anatomy and significant comorbidities that preclude open surgery. A prerequisite for a fenestrated cuff implantation must be experience in the planning and implantation of fenestrated aortic stent grafts; this places further limitations on the applicability of these devices.

There are several reports of the use of embolic and thrombus-inducing agents in the treatment of proximal type 1 endoleaks. Coil embolization of a proximal endoleak is achievable but the high pressure of the endoleak may cause recanalization over time. Endoleaks have also been treated by n-butyl cyanoacrylate (n-BCA) which is a clear free-flowing liquid which polymerizes into a solid material when in contact with anionic inhibitors found in excess in the blood. Solid n-BCA is attractive because it has a good chance of sealing a high-flow leak without the likelihood of recanalization. There is the risk of distal embolization when using n-BCA, and for this reason some advocate the combined transarterial use of coils and n-BCA.

One final discussion point is the coexistence of the type 2 endoleak. The continued pressurization due to type 2 endoleak may lead to aneurysm expansion and threaten the seal zones. It is possible that a persistent type 2 endoleak may be a precursor to a proximal type 1 endoleak in some patients. This has implications for the selection of patients for treatment of type 2 endoleaks.

Tips

- Proximal type 1 endoleaks are associated with a risk of aneurysm rupture.
- Understanding the precise etiology of the endoleak is crucial when defining treatment.
- Implantation of a proximal aortic cuff is a common treatment option for proximal type 1 endoleaks but may lead to compromise of the renal blood supply and may only work in around half of patients.

Commentary

Proximal type 1 (Type 1a) endoleaks post EVAR should be treated whether they occur early or late. The authors have discussed the various treatment options available in the preceding section.

The majority of patients can be managed by either insertion of an aortic cuff (where there is space between the renal arteries and the upper margin of the graft material) or by a supporting Palmaz stent to improve the seal between the endograft and aortic neck (if there is no space).

Fenestrated cuffs can be used if the above options fail or cannot be used, although as mentioned above, insertion of these devices is challenging, more so than the insertion of conventional fenestrated aortic endografts. Embolization has a role if none of the above measures work or cannot be used. In addition to coils and glue, onyx is also a useful embolic agent to consider.

Finally, in the presence of a type 1a endoleak, patent lumbar arteries may act as outflow vessels for the endoleak rather than inflow vessels. At this time, intervention for type 2 endoleaks is only indicated if there is evidence of aneurysm sac enlargement. Embolization is the treatment of choice and can be achieved either by the transarterial or percutaneous translumbar route.

Further Reading

Adam DJ, Fitridge RA, Berce M, Hartley DE, Anderson JL. Salvage of failed prior endovascular abdominal aortic aneurysm repair with fenestrated endovascular stent graft. J Vasc Surg. 2006;44:1341–4.

Becquemin JP, Kelley L, Zubilewicz T, et al. Outcomes of secondary interventions after abdominal aortic aneurysm endovascular repair. J Vasc Surg. 2004;39:298–305.

Maldonado TS, Rosen RJ, Rockman CB, et al. Initial successful management of type I endoleak after endovascular aortic aneurysm repair with n-butyl cyanoacrylate adhesive. J Vasc Surg. 2003;38:664–70.

Peynircioulu B, Türkbey B, Özkan M, et al. Use of glue and microcoils for transarterial catheter embolization of a type 1 endoleak. Diagn Interv Radiol. 2008;14:111–5.

Stefandis D, Chiou AC, Kashyap V, Toursarkissian B. Treatment of a late-appearing proximal type-1 endoleak after Ancure graft with an AneuRx cuff – a case report. Vasc Endovascular Surg. 2003;37(6): 437–40.

Chapter 17
Management of a Type 1B Endoleak Following EVAR

Robert P. Allison, Anna Maria Belli, Joo-Young Chun, Raymond Chung, Raj Das, Andrew England, Karen Flood, Marie-France Giroux, Richard G. McWilliams, Robert Morgan, Nik Papadakos, Jai V. Patel, Raf Patel, Uday Patel, Lakshmi Ratnam, Reddi Prasad Yadavali, and John Rose

Abstract This case reviews the management of a distal type 1 endoleak following EVAR by embolization of the internal iliac artery. Displacement of a coil during the procedure is also discussed.

Keywords Complications • EVAR • Type 1 endoleak • Embolization • Coil displacement

---

R.P. Allison
Department of Interventional Radiology, University Hospitals Southampton, Southampton, Hampshire, UK

A.M. Belli
Department of Radiology, St. George's Hospital and Medical School, Blackshaw Road, London SW17 0RE, UK
e-mail: anna.belli@stgeorges.nhs.uk

J.-Y. Chun • R. Chung • R. Das
R. Morgan • N. Papadakos
Department of Radiology, St. George's Hospital, London, UK

A. England
Department of Radiography, University of Salford, Manchester, UK

K. Flood
Department of Vascular Radiology, Leeds General Infirmary,
Leeds, UK

M.-F. Giroux
Department of Radiology, CHUM-Centre Hospitalier
de l'Université de Montréal, Montreal, QC, Canada

R.G. McWilliams
Department of Radiology, Royal Liverpool University Hospital,
Liverpool, UK

J.V. Patel
Department of Radiology, The Leeds Teaching Hospitals NHS Trust,
Leeds, West Yorkshire, UK

R. Patel
Department of Radiology,
The Leeds Teaching Hospitals NHS Trust,
Leeds, West Yorkshire, UK
e-mail: rafpatel@gmail.com

U. Patel
Department of Diagnostic Radiology, St. George's Hospital and
Medical School, Blackshaw Road, SW17 0QT London, UK
e-mail: uday.patel@stgeorges.nhs.uk

L. Ratnam
Department of Radiology, St. George's Hospital, Blackshaw Road,
SW17 0QT London, UK
e-mail: lakshmi.ratnam@nhs.net

R.P. Yadavali
Department of Radiology, Aberdeen Royal Infirmary, Aberdeen, UK

J. Rose
Department of Interventional Radiology, Freeman Hospital,
Newcastle Upon Tyne Hospitals NHS Trust, Newcastle upon Tyne, UK

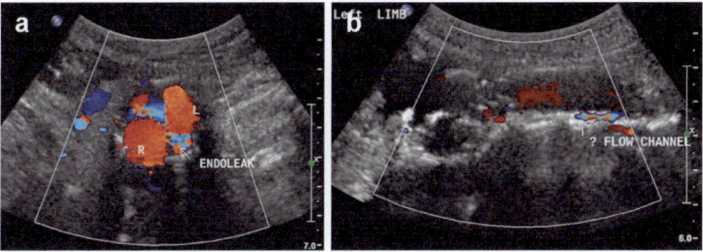

FIGURE 17.1 (**a**) Doppler ultrasound demonstrating blood flow both within the aneurysm and the endoleak between the two iliac limbs (*arrow*); (**b**) Doppler ultrasound demonstrating blood flow between the left iliac limb and the posterior wall of the common iliac artery (*arrow*) suggesting that the endoleak is a distal type 1

Case History

An 82-year-old man underwent elective EVAR for a 7.7 cm AAA using a Gore bifurcated device (W. L. Gore & Associates, Flagstaff, AZ). After graft deployment there was a proximal type 1 endoleak which resolved following moulding with a Coda balloon (Cook Inc, Bloomington, IN).

Follow-up arterial phase CT, in another center, revealed the presence of a large endoleak of unknown etiology. Doppler ultrasound demonstrated a large endoleak in the distal aneurysm (Fig. 17.1a) with a track along the posterior aspect of the distal left limb (Fig. 17.1b). Contrast-enhanced ultrasound (CEUS) was performed, and this demonstrated the simultaneous appearance of contrast medium in the stent graft and the aneurysm sac around the distal stent graft. These appearances were consistent with a distal type 1 endoleak. Arrangements were made for urgent endovascular treatment of the leak.

Procedure

Ultrasound-guided puncture of the left common femoral artery was performed following administration of prophylactic antibiotics. Angiography with direct injection into the left

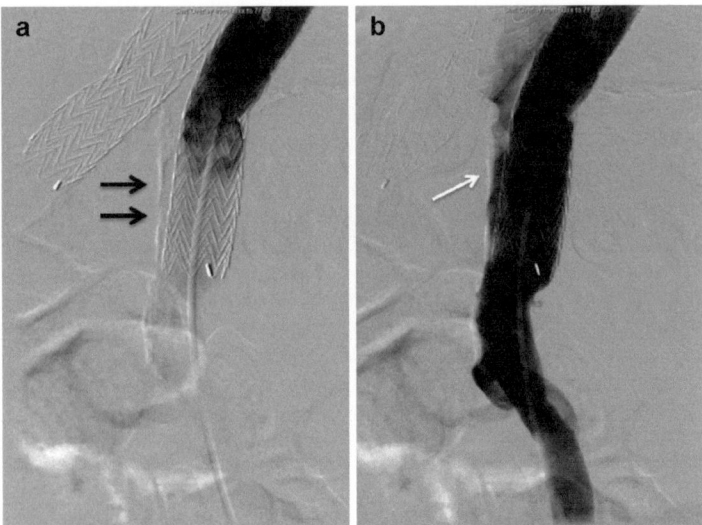

Figure 17.2 (**a**) The distal type 1 endoleak is the result of incomplete apposition of the iliac limb against the calcified common iliac artery wall (*arrows*); (**b**) high frame rate angiogram demonstrating retrograde flow of contrast (*white arrow*) into the aneurysm sac from a gap between the iliac limb and common iliac artery wall

iliac limb demonstrated a large distal type 1 endoleak. Furthermore, there was incomplete apposition of the original iliac limb against the common iliac artery wall (Fig. 17.2a). A high frame rate angiographic run showed filling of the endoleak before the lumbar arteries filled via the internal iliac (Fig. 17.2b). This confirmed the endoleak to be a type 1B rather than a lumbar type 2. The left internal iliac artery was embolized with three 12 mm embolization coils. One of the coils hooked on the catheter as it was removed and displaced proximally although the coil did not migrate into the external iliac artery (Fig. 17.3). Following this a 16-13-93 Endurant iliac limb extension (Medtronic, Santa Rosa, CA) was placed into the Gore limb on the left side and extended into the left external iliac artery. After first release, there was still some flow between the stent-graft limbs which allowed continued

Chapter 17. Type 1B Endoleak Following EVAR   125

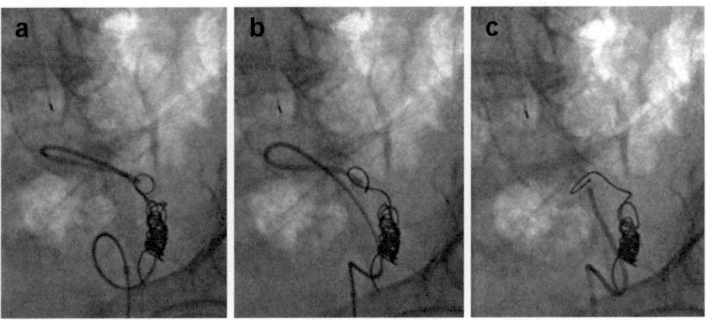

FIGURE 17.3 A sequence of fluoroscopy images following deployment of the embolization coils. The most proximal coil is caught on the catheter tip. Shaking and manipulating the catheter finally releases the embolization coil

perfusion of the internal iliac artery. A 16 mm angioplasty balloon was inflated at the junction between the two limbs, and a further 12 mm angioplasty balloon was used to dilate the external iliac artery. Completion angiography confirmed exclusion of the endoleak and good flow into the iliac system (Fig. 17.4).

Discussion

An endoleak is the presence of blood flow outside the lumen of the stent graft and is classified according to the system devised by White and May in 1997. A distal type 1 endoleak (type 1B) occurs when a persistent channel of blood develops due to an inadequate seal at the distal margins of the device. The reported incidence of type 1 endoleaks ranges from 0 to 10 % and presents more frequently in patients with short, calcified, ectatic, and tortuous common iliac arteries. Distal type 1 endoleaks are also generally associated with a greater number of adverse events, and although some endoleaks resolve spontaneously, it is difficult to predict and a large proportion will require early reintervention. Review of data

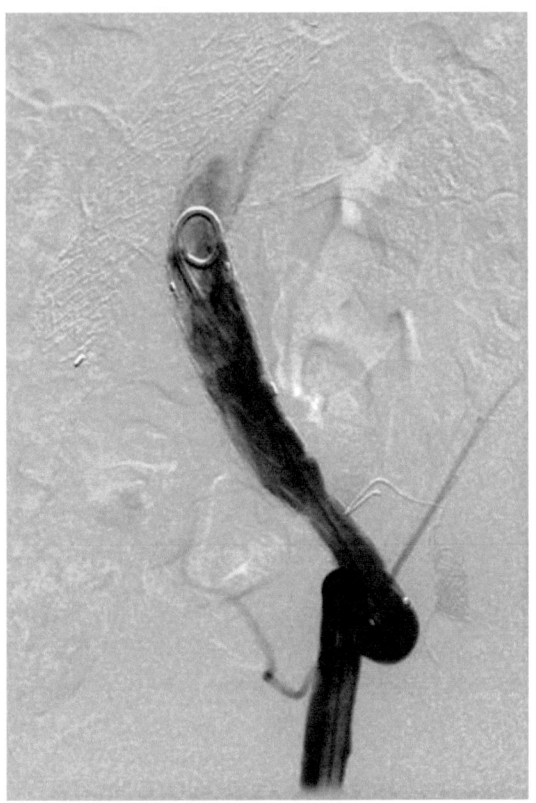

Figure 17.4 Angiography following embolization and implantation of the iliac extension. There has been total resolution of the distal type 1 endoleak, and there is absence of any blood flow in the internal iliac artery

from the EUROSTAR registry concludes that distal type 1 endoleaks are independent risk factors for late conversion to open repair (risk ratio 2.61 95 % CI 1.29–5.28).

Ideally distal type 1 endoleaks should be prevented by careful sizing of the iliac limbs and by ensuring sufficient coverage of the common iliac artery upon deployment. If this is not the case, then treatment options include balloon remodelling of the attachment site or extension of the stent graft into the distal common iliac or external iliac arteries. If the latter is the case and if the origin of the internal iliac artery needs to be covered, then this should be embolized first using coils to prevent retrograde endoleak. This is not necessarily a benign procedure. Some reports have documented a 28 % risk of buttock claudication post-embolization of the internal iliac artery, while others have reported a much lower incidence of adverse events.

Deployment of a Palmaz stent (Cordis, Miami, FL) can also be an effective method for achieving a seal, especially if the endoleak results from regional infolding of the stent graft. The use of a balloon-expandable uncovered stent will however not be effective if the original stent-graft limb was undersized. Alternatively and less frequently, embolization of the endoleak using coils or liquid embolic agents can be achieved. In the majority of cases, early or late distal type 1 endoleaks are treated by distal extension of the endograft. Conversion to open aortic repair should only be considered in the presence of an associated stent-graft infection, if endovascular reintervention fails or if there is continued aneurysm growth without any further identifiable endoleaks.

With the potential for delayed (late) type 1 distal endoleaks, lifelong imaging surveillance after EVAR is considered necessary. The majority of these late endoleaks can be successfully treated by endovascular reinterventions and complex open aortic surgery avoided.

Tips

- Distal type 1 endoleaks can occur early or late following EVAR.
- Careful preoperative sizing of the distal components together with coverage of a long segment of the common iliac artery reduces the risk of endoleak.
- If a distal type 1 endoleak exists, prompt treatment is recommended, and for the majority, this is by an endovascular approach.

- Extension of an iliac limb into the external iliac artery combined with coil embolization of the internal iliac artery is an effective treatment. There is a risk of associated buttock claudication, and assessment of the contribution to pelvic perfusion from both internal iliac arteries should be considered before this type of reintervention.

Commentary

The best strategy to avoid the complication described here is to ensure that a long length of the common iliac artery is covered by the stent graft, but once this has occurred, the solution described by the authors is the most practical. Although covering a patent artery is better avoided, even bilateral occlusion of the internal iliac arteries can be safely performed particularly when proximal coils or plugs are used, leaving the branches patent for reperfusion by collaterals.

Further Reading

Bratby MJ, Munneke GM, Belli AM, Loosemore TM, Loftus I, Thompson MM, Morgan RA. How safe is bilateral internal iliac embolization prior to EVAR? Cardiovasc Intervent Radiol. 2008;31:246–53.

Liaw JVP, Clark M, Gibbs R, Jenkins M, Cheshire N, Hamady M. Update: complications and management of infrarenal EVAR. Eur J Radiol. 2009;71:541–51.

Rayt HS, Bown MJ, Lambert KV, Fishwick NG, McCarthy MJ, London NJ. Buttock claudication and erectile dysfunction after internal iliac artery embolization in patients prior to endovascular aortic aneurysm repair. Cardiovasc Intervent Radiol. 2008;31(4):728–34.

Vallabhaneni SR, Harris PL. Lessons learnt from the EUROSTAR registry on endovascular repair of abdominal aortic aneurysm repair. Eur J Radiol. 2001;39:34–41.

Chapter 18
Persistent Type 2 Endoleak Post-EVAR with Aneurysm Expansion

Robert P. Allison, Anna Maria Belli, Joo-Young Chun, Raymond Chung, Raj Das, Andrew England, Karen Flood, Marie-France Giroux, Richard G. McWilliams, Robert Morgan, Nik Papadakos, Jai V. Patel, Raf Patel, Uday Patel, Lakshmi Ratnam, Reddi Prasad Yadavali, and John Rose

Abstract This case illustrates the treatment of a type 2 endoleak following fenestrated EVAR by coil embolization of the IMA.

Keywords Complications • EVAR • Type 2 endoleak • Embolization • IMA

R.P. Allison
Department of Interventional Radiology, University Hospitals Southampton, Southampton, Hampshire, UK

A.M. Belli
Department of Radiology, St. George's Hospital and Medical School, Blackshaw Road, London SW17 0RE, UK
e-mail: anna.belli@stgeorges.nhs.uk

J.-Y. Chun • R. Chung • R. Das
R. Morgan • N. Papadakos
Department of Radiology, St. George's Hospital, London, UK

A. England
Department of Radiography, University of Salford,
Manchester, UK

K. Flood
Department of Vascular Radiology, Leeds General Infirmary,
Leeds, UK

M.-F. Giroux
Department of Radiology, CHUM-Centre Hospitalier de
l'Université de Montréal, Montreal, QC, Canada

R.G. McWilliams
Department of Radiology, Royal Liverpool University Hospital,
Liverpool, UK

J.V. Patel
Department of Radiology, The Leeds Teaching Hospitals NHS
Trust, Leeds, West Yorkshire, UK

R. Patel
Department of Radiology,
The Leeds Teaching Hospitals NHS Trust,
Leeds, West Yorkshire, UK
e-mail: rafpatel@gmail.com

U. Patel
Department of Diagnostic Radiology, St. George's Hospital
and Medical School, Blackshaw Road, SW17 0QT London, UK
e-mail: uday.patel@stgeorges.nhs.uk

L. Ratnam
Department of Radiology, St. George's Hospital, Blackshaw Road,
SW17 0QT London, UK
e-mail: lakshmi.ratnam@nhs.net

R.P. Yadavali
Department of Radiology, Aberdeen Royal Infirmary,
Aberdeen, UK

J. Rose
Department of Interventional Radiology, Freeman Hospital,
Newcastle Upon Tyne Hospitals NHS Trust,
Newcastle upon Tyne, UK

Chapter 18. Persistent Type 2 Endoleak Post-EVAR

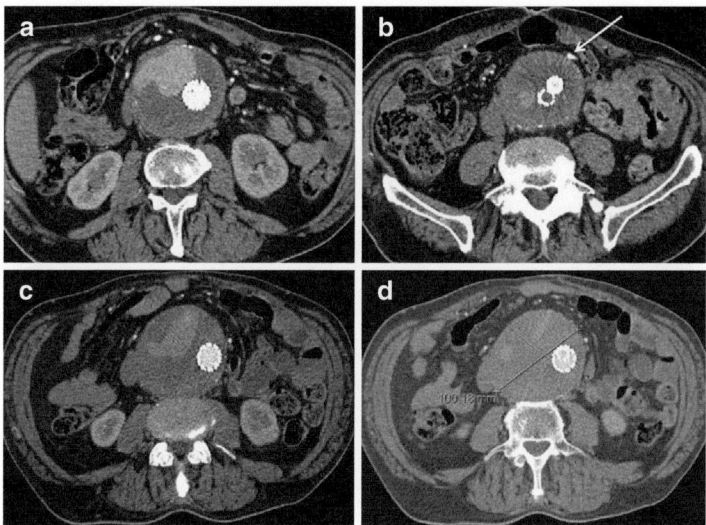

FIGURE 18.1 (**a**) 1st postoperative (1-month) CT scan showing a large type 2 endoleak; (**b**) 1st postoperative (1-month) CT scan showing a patent IMA (*arrow*). Incidentally there has been occlusion of the right iliac limb; (**c**) 6-month postoperative CT scan showing persistence of the large type 2 endoleak; (**d**) with further expansion of the aneurysm

Case History

A 78-year-old man presented with an 8.8-cm asymptomatic juxtarenal AAA and was referred for fenestrated endovascular aortic aneurysm repair (FEVAR). Following the implantation, a large type 2 endoleak was demonstrated on the 1-month baseline CT scan (Fig. 18.1a). Contrast medium was also seen in the inferior mesenteric artery (IMA) which lay in close proximity to the aneurysm sac (Fig. 18.1b). Six months later the endoleak was still present (Fig. 18.1c), the right limb of the graft had occluded, and the aneurysm had expanded to 10 cm (Fig. 18.1d). With the presence of both an endoleak and continued expansion of the aneurysm, the patient was scheduled for a catheter angiogram with a view to treating the endoleak.

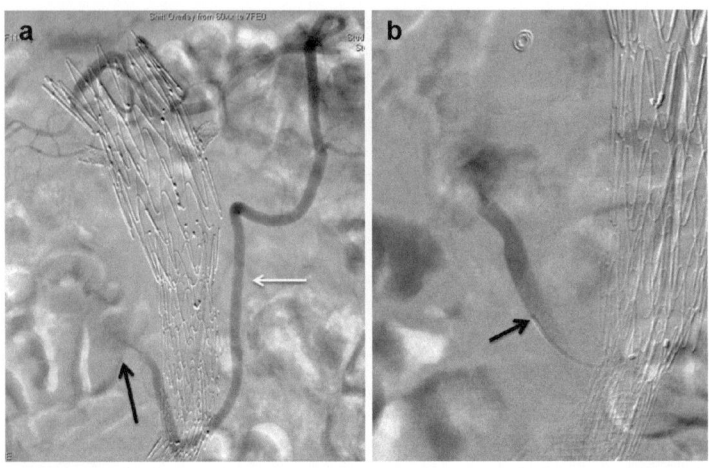

Figure 18.2 (a) Selective SMA angiogram (early phase) demonstrating the type 2 endoleak (*black arrow*) fed by the IMA via the arc of Riolan (*white arrow*); (b) the microcatheter was positioned in the stem of the IMA (*arrow*) prior to the deployment of the Vortex embolization coils

Procedure

Ultrasound-guided access of the left common femoral artery was performed. A superior mesenteric artery (SMA) angiogram confirmed a large type 2 endoleak fed by the IMA via the arc of Riolan (Fig. 18.2a). A triple coaxial system was used to gain access; a sheath was fed into the proximal SMA, a 5-Fr catheter into the middle colic artery, and then a Progreat microcatheter (Terumo Medical Corp, Somerset, NJ), after this. The microcatheter was taken through to the origin of the IMA (Fig. 18.2b). Estimations from the CT scans suggested that 4-mm coils would be suitable and nondetachable 4-mm Vortex coils (Boston Scientific, Natick, MA) were used (Fig. 18.3a). These formed well in the IMA although the first coil was carried by flow into the aneurysm. As the microcatheter was withdrawn, the coil nest was pulled back to the level of the division of the IMA into the left colic, sigmoid, and superior rectal branches (Fig. 18.3b). The coils were pushed back into the IMA stem with a guidewire; 5-mm coils were

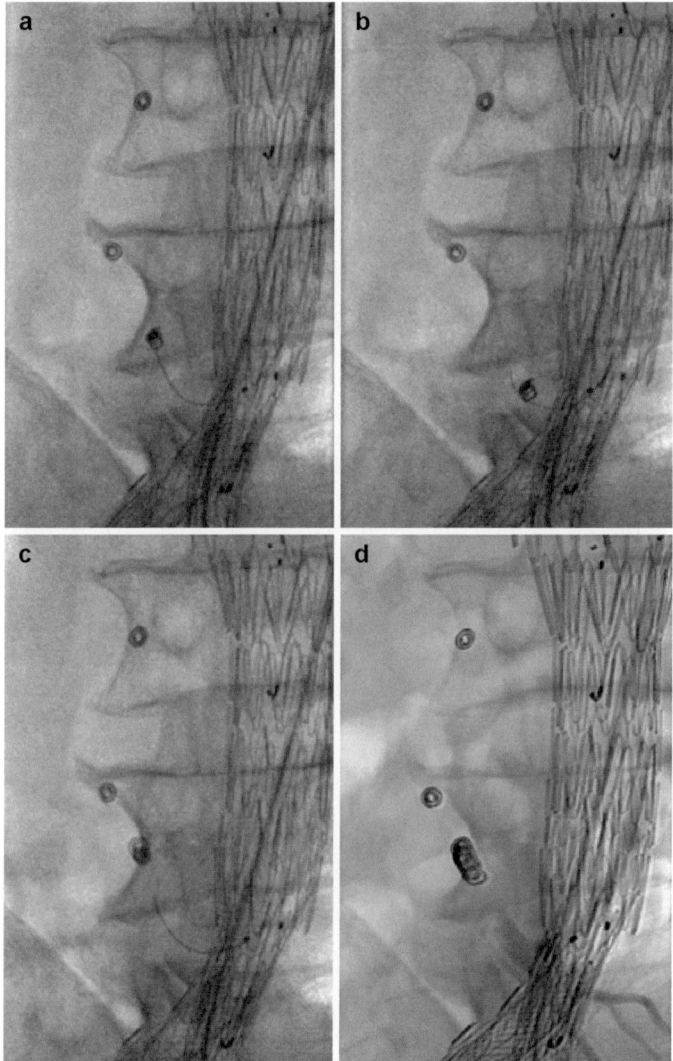

FIGURE 18.3 (**a**) Following deployment of the 4-mm Vortex coils, the coil nest was inadvertently pulled back to the level of the division of the IMA into the left colic, sigmoid, and superior rectal branches as the microcatheter was withdrawn (**b**, **c**) the coils were pushed back into the IMA stem with a guidewire; (**d**) 5-mm coils were then placed behind the 4-mm coils

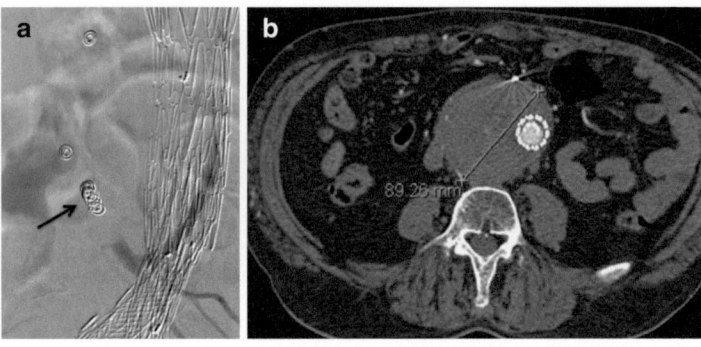

FIGURE 18.4 (**a**) Angiogram following deployment of the embolization coils (*arrow*). There is now absence of blood flow with the aneurysm sac; (**b**) follow-up CT scan at 2 years showing absence of the type 2 endoleak and reduction in the size of the aneurysm

then placed behind the 4-mm coils (Fig. 18.3c, d). A final angiogram showed complete absence of blood flow into the aneurysm sac (Fig. 18.4a). Follow-up CT at 14 months confirmed that the aneurysm had been successfully excluded. A further CT at 2 years again confirmed that the aneurysm was excluded and that it had shrunk down to 8.9 cm in maximum diameter (Fig. 18.4b).

Discussion

Type 2 endoleaks are common and are reported in approximately 20–30 % of EVAR patients during follow-up. They may occur at any time and the majority have a negligible effect on aneurysm rupture risk, and around 80 % will resolve spontaneously. However, not all type II endoleaks are harmless, and there is evidence that they are associated with aneurysm expansion and secondary reinterventions. Some clinicians advocate treatment if a type 2 endoleak has persisted for more than 6 months. However, most operators recommend intervention for type 2 endoleaks if there is documented expansion of the aneurysm sac. The amount of expansion before considering treatment varies between different centers.

Definitive treatment includes transarterial and translumbar embolization using coils or liquid embolic agents, laparoscopic or open ligation of the relevant feeding vessels, and open surgical conversion. The most common management technique is transfemoral embolization of the feeding vessels. The principle of this treatment is to eliminate the feeding branches at their junction with the aneurysm. Initial results for catheter embolization are favorable, but selective catheterization of feeding vessels may be technically challenging. Transarterial embolization can have a relatively high failure rate of up to 80 %. It is possible that multiple patent collateral arteries allow both inflow and outflow of blood from the aneurysm sac. This may lead to the persistence of a type 2 endoleak despite coil embolization. Reports have documented the development of additional endoleaks even after apparently successful coil embolization warranting further repeat reinterventions.

Translumbar embolization is another technique where a needle is advanced into the endoleak cavity usually under CT guidance. The patient is then transferred to the interventional suite where angiography is performed followed by coil embolization. Translumbar embolization can be offered as primary treatment or after transarterial failure. Translumbar techniques have been suggested as being more durable with >90 % success being maintained after 8 months. Mansueto et al. have shown promising results from a transcaval embolization route for type 2 endoleaks. Aneurysm sac puncture is performed through the inferior vena cava, and an embolic agent is injected into the aneurysm sac until there is no more evidence of blood flow. Intrasac pressure measurements can be used to confirm successful embolization and full exclusion of the aneurysm. Early results have suggested that this procedure is comparable with translumbar embolization. Embolic agents other than coils can also be used and include Onyx, Ethibloc, thrombin, and cyanoacrylate.

Laparoscopic peritoneal ligation is another option. This involves the surgical ligation of the inferior mesenteric and lumbar arteries. A further possibility is a surgical sac fenestration where the aneurysm sac is opened, thrombus removed, and back-bleeding vessels oversewn while leaving the stent graft in place. Open surgical conversion should only be offered in exceptional cases where less-invasive options are not appropriate or have failed and where the aneurysm is large and growing.

The visualization of a patent IMA on preoperative imaging has been associated with late type 2 endoleaks. With this in mind, consideration has been given to the benefits of prophylactic embolization before or during the EVAR procedure. Such interventions have, however, provided no reduction in the number of type 2 endoleaks. Finally, when evaluating a patient with a type 2 endoleak, a risk-benefit analysis should be conducted comparing close follow-up versus early intervention and should take into account the age of the patient, AAA size, vessels involved, and the expected efficacy of any treatment.

Tips

- Patients with a large patent IMA or more than two lumbar arteries on preoperative CT are at increased risk for developing a type 2 endoleak.
- There is no clear evidence to justify pre- or intraoperative embolization of the IMA or lumbar arteries.
- A type 2 endoleak in a stable or regressing aneurysm can be safely treated with conservative management.
- Catheter-based embolization techniques should be the first treatment option for type 2 endoleaks in expanding aneurysms.
- Endoleaks may recur and additional repeat interventional procedures may be required.
- Complex endoleaks which involve multiple inflow/outflow collaterals may not be amenable to either embolization or laparoscopic ligation.

Commentary

This case demonstrates successful embolization of the inferior mesenteric artery from the superior mesenteric artery in the treatment of a type 2 endoleak associated with expansion of the aneurysm sac.

In general, the evidence that type 2 endoleaks are associated with late aneurysm rupture and death is very limited, although most authors consider that sac expansion is dangerous and recommend treatment of the type 2 endoleak if this occurs.

The jury is out on the relative merits of transarterial versus translumbar embolization routes. There are proponents of both techniques and in most centers; the choice of technique comes down to individual preference. Very little evidence is available showing that successful embolization (by either route) is durable and effective in preventing further sac expansion and late aneurysm rupture.

Clearly, there is a lot of scope for research in this sphere to answer the above important questions.

Further Reading

Buth J, Harris PL, Van Marrewijk C, Fransen G. Endoleaks during follow-up after endovascular repair of abdominal aortic aneurysm. Are they all dangerous? J Cardiovasc Surg (Torino). 2003;44(4):559–66.

Jones JE, Atkins MD, Brewster DC, Chung TK, Kwolek CJ, LaMuraglia GM. Persistent type 2 endoleak after endovascular repair of abdominal aortic aneurysm is associated with adverse late outcomes. J Vasc Surg. 2007;46:1–8.

Jonker FHW, Aruny J, Muhs BE. Management of type II endoleaks: preoperative versus postoperative versus expectant management. Semin Vasc Surg. 2009;22:165–71.

Mansueto G, Cenzi D, Scuro A, Gottin L, Griso A, Gumbs AA, et al. Treatment of type II endoleak with a transcatheter transcaval approach: results at 1-year follow-up. J Vasc Surg. 2007;45(6):1120–7.

van Marrewijk CJ, Fransen G, Laheij RJF, Harris PL, Buth J, EUROSTAR Collaborators. Is a type II endoleak after EVAR a harbinger of risk? Causes and outcome of open conversion and aneurysm rupture during follow-up. Eur J Vasc Endovasc Surg. 2004;27:128–37.

Chapter 19
Acute Renal Artery Occlusion and Trapped Renal Artery Catheter During Infrarenal AAA Stent Grafting

Robert P. Allison, Anna Maria Belli, Joo-Young Chun, Raymond Chung, Raj Das, Andrew England, Karen Flood, Marie-France Giroux, Richard G. McWilliams, Robert Morgan, Nik Papadakos, Jai V. Patel, Raf Patel, Uday Patel, Lakshmi Ratnam, Reddi Prasad Yadavali, and John Rose

Abstract This case reviews the management of an occluded renal artery by the fabric of an aortic stent graft during an EVAR procedure.

Keywords Complications • EVAR • Renal artery occlusion • Balloon-expandable stent

R.P. Allison
Department of Interventional Radiology, University Hospitals Southampton, Southampton, Hampshire, UK

A.M. Belli
Department of Radiology, St. George's Hospital and Medical School, Blackshaw Road, London SW17 0RE, UK
e-mail: anna.belli@stgeorges.nhs.uk

J.-Y. Chun • R. Chung • R. Das
R. Morgan • N. Papadakos
Department of Radiology, St. George's Hospital, London, UK

A. England
Department of Radiography, University of Salford, Manchester, UK

K. Flood
Department of Vascular Radiology, Leeds General Infirmary,
Leeds, UK

M.-F. Giroux
Department of Radiology, CHUM-Centre Hospitalier
de l'Université de Montréal, Montreal, QC, Canada

R.G. McWilliams
Department of Radiology, Royal Liverpool University Hospital,
Liverpool, UK

J.V. Patel
Department of Radiology, The Leeds Teaching Hospitals NHS Trust,
Leeds, West Yorkshire, UK

R. Patel
Department of Radiology,
The Leeds Teaching Hospitals NHS Trust,
Leeds, West Yorkshire, UK
e-mail: rafpatel@gmail.com

U. Patel
Department of Diagnostic Radiology, St. George's Hospital and
Medical School, Blackshaw Road, SW17 0QT London, UK
e-mail: uday.patel@stgeorges.nhs.uk

L. Ratnam
Department of Radiology, St. George's Hospital, Blackshaw Road,
SW17 0QT London, UK
e-mail: lakshmi.ratnam@nhs.net

R.P. Yadavali
Department of Radiology, Aberdeen Royal Infirmary, Aberdeen, UK

J. Rose
Department of Interventional Radiology, Freeman Hospital,
Newcastle Upon Tyne Hospitals NHS Trust, Newcastle upon Tyne, UK

Chapter 19. Renal Artery Occlusion During EVAR

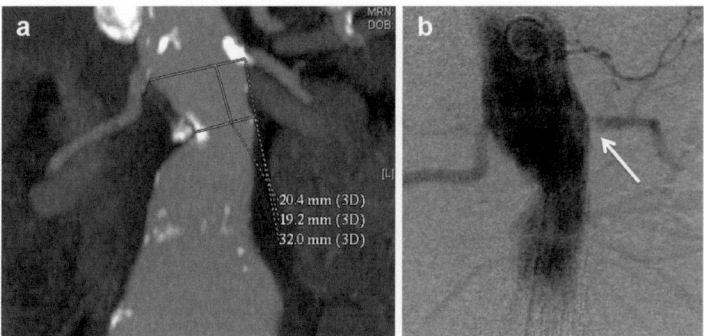

Figure 19.1 (**a**) Coronal CT reformatted image demonstrating a short reverse conical aortic neck and patent bilateral renal arteries; (**b**) initial completion angiogram demonstrating fabric coverage over the origin of the left renal artery (*arrow*)

Case History

A 75-year-old man was referred with an asymptomatic abdominal aortic aneurysm (AAA). Preoperative CT scanning confirmed a 7.8 cm infrarenal AAA with a short and reversed conical aortic neck (Fig. 19.1a). The patient underwent an elective endovascular repair (EVAR) with implantation of a Zenith bifurcated device (Cook INC, Bloomington, IN). The main body of the Zenith device was deployed from the right common femoral artery. Angiography post-deployment demonstrated fabric coverage of the left renal artery ostium (Fig. 19.1b). Unsuccessful attempts were then made to manually displace the stent graft inferiorly. The reversed taper of the infrarenal neck prevented caudal displacement of the fabric. A decision was made to stent the left renal artery.

Procedure

A reversed curve catheter was positioned in the upper abdominal aorta and the left renal artery catheterized with some difficulty. Attempted withdrawal of the catheter was seen to

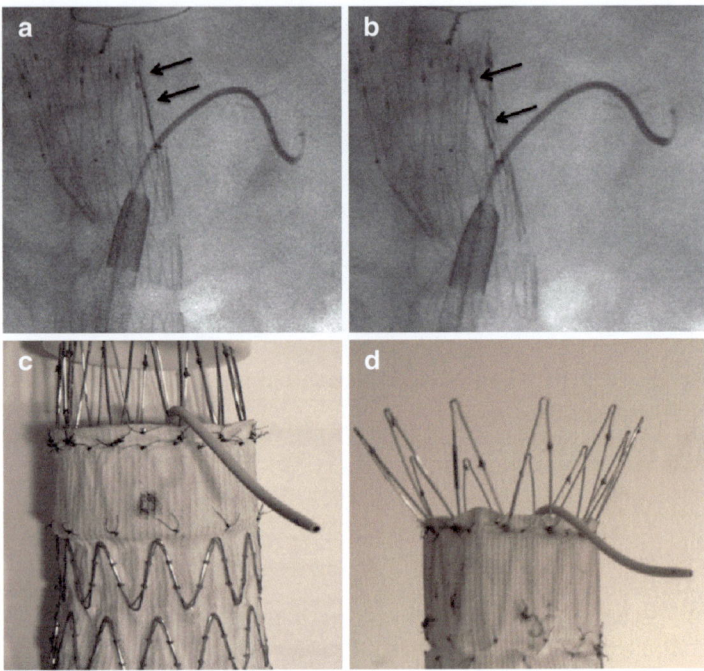

FIGURE 19.2 (**a**) Reverse curve catheter "wedged" in the inferior apex of the bare anchor stent. (**b**) The radiopaque marker strut (*arrows*) can be seen to move medially when an attempt is made to withdraw the catheter (**c, d**) photographs illustrating the radiological appearances in (**a, c**). The catheter is "wedged" in the inferior portion of the V in the bare suprarenal stent; the inferior portion of the V is tighter when the stent graft is constrained within the aortic lumen; (**d**) the degree of catheter wedging at the V is reduced when the stent graft is not constrained within the abdominal aorta

deform the anchor stent pulling struts medially (Fig. 19.2a). The catheter appeared to be wedged at the base of the anchor stent where the wireforms create a narrow "V" (Fig. 19.2b). In order to remove the catheter from its trapped position, a sheath was introduced and passed over the catheter in order to help elevate it during retraction (Fig. 19.3a). This technique was successful, and both a guidewire and catheter were then

Chapter 19. Renal Artery Occlusion During EVAR 143

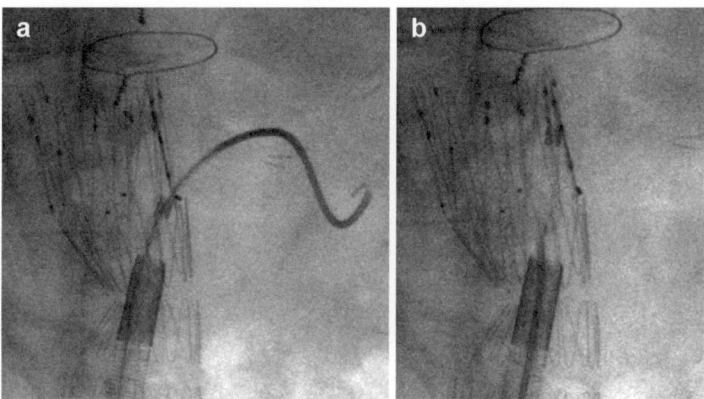

FIGURE 19.3 (**a**) A sheath has been used to elevate and successfully free the wedged catheter; (**b**) the catheter and guidewire are now within the stent graft in the aortic lumen and can be advanced through the larger spaces between the stent struts and into the left renal artery

successfully introduced into the left renal artery through the larger space between stent struts (Fig. 19.3b). Following this a 6×17 mm Palmaz Genesis balloon-expandable stent (Cordis, Miami, FL) was deployed into the left renal artery (Fig. 19.4a). Good renal blood flow was reestablished and the patient made an uneventful recovery and was discharged home.

Discussion

A secure proximal seal is an absolute requirement for successful EVAR. A short aortic neck often excludes many patients from infrarenal EVAR, and for those where treatment is considered, deployment of the stent graft in close proximity to the renal artery ostia is essential. Accurate device positioning can be problematic in the presence of an angulated neck. If inadvertent coverage of a renal artery ostium does occur, then this may be serious. Early identification of inadvertent coverage is essential as are the skills necessary to deal with this problem.

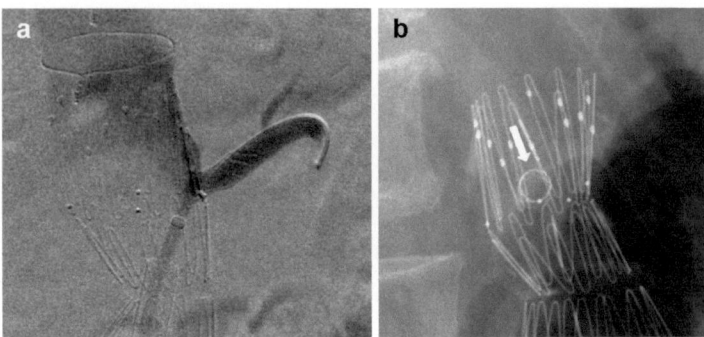

Figure 19.4 (**a**) Angiogram post-deployment of a balloon-expandable stent. Good flow has now been restored to the left renal artery; (**b**) lateral abdominal radiograph confirming that the bare renal stent has been deployed through the widest V space (*arrow*) of the bare suprarenal anchor stent

Reports within the literature document a 1 % renal artery occlusion rate following EVAR. The incidence of renal infarction is higher at 1.5 %, and this figure undoubtedly takes into account the intentional occlusion of accessory renal arteries. The unintentional placement of the fabric portion of the stent graft across a renal artery ostium can increase the risk of renal failure, loss of functional renal parenchyma, renovascular hypertension, and dialysis dependency. Reports of cases where there has been coverage of a single main renal artery suggest that this complication may result in deterioration in renal function; possible worsening of hypertension but overall patients should be spared dialysis.

Mechanical displacement of the stent graft by caudal traction may be attempted initially. The decision to attempt this will depend on the clinical situation, stent graft used, and the stage of deployment when renal coverage is noted. If renal artery coverage is noted before full release of the stent graft from its ipsilateral attachment, then controlled caudal traction on the delivery system may provide enough fabric displacement to allow full reperfusion of the affected renal artery and alleviate the need for any additional interventions (Fig. 19.5). Displacement is also

Chapter 19. Renal Artery Occlusion During EVAR 145

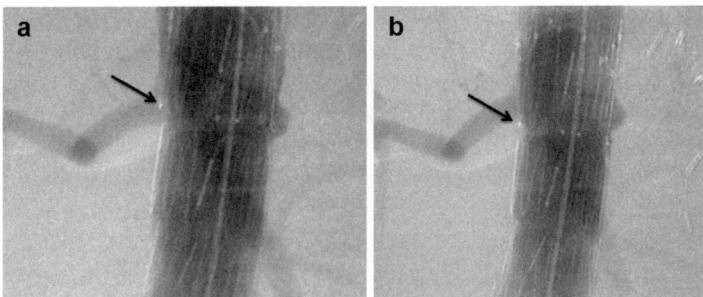

FIGURE 19.5 (**a**) Intraoperative aortogram demonstrating partial coverage of the right renal ostium (*fabric marker marked with arrow*), the patient has also had a previous left nephrectomy; (**b**) at this point in the procedure, the stent graft had not been completely deployed; as a result it was possible to manually distract the aortic stent graft distally and resolve the renal artery coverage (arrow shows fabric marker now lies below the right renal ostium)

reported to be possible by crossing the stent-graft bifurcation with a guidewire and retrieving this using a snare from the contralateral groin. A catheter must then traverse the guidewire and be exteriorized in both groins. A displacement force can then be applied which can move the main body of the device caudally and restore flow to the affected renal artery. Similar results have also been described using a balloon inflated within the main body of the stent graft and manually distracted.

If manual traction fails and the degree of renal artery coverage is small, access to the renal artery either by the transfemoral or transbrachial routes is rarely difficult. A stent can then be placed within the ostium of the compromised renal artery to restore perfusion. The choice of whether to deploy a bare or covered stent is a matter of personal preference. It is our practice to use balloon-expandable bare stents for the treatment of fabric encroachment of renal artery ostia. If severe coverage exists, renal artery access may only be achievable via a brachial approach. The short- and medium-term primary patency rates for renal artery stents are excellent following EVAR, and this adds to the evidence for their use prior to any more invasive bailouts.

Surgical extra-anatomical revascularization is also a potential treatment option for acute occlusion of a renal artery and is achievable by the hepatorenal, splenorenal, iliorenal, and thoracic aortorenal routes. Surgical conversion to open repair is also a consideration; however, this is challenging in the presence of a deployed stent graft. High mortality rates have been associated with elective conversions to open repair. However, there are reports within the literature describing open conversion in the face of inadvertent renal artery coverage.

Finally, fluoroscopic guidance of EVAR procedures is not free from errors. Projectional errors can arise and have a resultant effect on the deployment of a stent graft. Most clinicians routinely adjust the orientation of the c-arm in order to reflect the rotation and angulation of the renal arteries leaving the aorta. Several additional adjunctive measures have also been described in order to enhance proximal stent-graft deployment accuracy and to improve the identification of the most caudal renal artery. One approach involves leaving a catheter in the most caudal renal artery. The main body of the device can be deployed and then this catheter withdrawn.

Tips

- Poor renal artery visualization after stent-graft deployment may indicate coverage of the renal ostium by the fabric of the device.
- Renal artery stenting is a prompt method for dealing with inadvertent renal artery coverage if manual displacement fails or is not considered appropriate.
- The bare metal components of suprarenal stent grafts can act as a trap for catheters and guidewires.
- Steps should be employed to ensure that adjuvant renal artery stents are deployed through the widest sections of the bare suprarenal stent struts (Fig. 19.4b). When advancing a sheath through the bare stent into the renal artery, if there is resistance, then this may be an indicator that the catheter is trying to advance through the narrower V space and should be repositioned.

- Troubleshooting difficulty during EVAR is facilitated if the operator has the opportunity to assess a sample stent graft and delivery system in vitro.

Commentary

This case demonstrates how to deal with two related complications. Inadvertent coverage of the renal arteries should be recognized and remedied promptly. If the stent graft cannot be moved, then placing a stent into the renal artery is necessary. Catheterization and manipulation in renal arteries is not always straightforward, and good guidewire and catheter skills are essential to avoid further injury and improve chances of success.

Further Reading

Greenberg RK, Chuter TA, Lawrence-Brown M, Haulon S, Nolte L. Analysis of renal function after aneurysm repair with a device using suprarenal fixation (Zenith AAA Endovascular Graft) in contrast to open surgical repair. J Vasc Surg. 2004;39:1219–28.

Hiramoto JS, Chang CK, Reilly LM, Schneider DB, Rapp JH, Chuter TAM. Outcomes of renal stenting for renal artery coverage during endovascular aortic aneurysm repair. J Vasc Surg. 2009;49:1100–6.

Lin PH, Bush RL, Lumsden AB. Endovascular rescue of a maldeployed aortic stent-graft causing renal artery occlusion: technical considerations. Vasc Endovascular Surg. 2004;38:69–73.

Maher H, Geroulakos G, Hughes DA, Moser S, Shepherd A, Salama AD. Delayed hepato-spleno-renal bypass for renal salvage following malposition of an infrarenal aortic stent-graft. J Endovasc Ther. 2010;17(3):326–31.

Weinberger JB, Long GW, Bove PG, Uzieblo MR, Kirsch MJ, Richey KA, et al. Intentional coverage of a main renal artery during endovascular juxtarenal aortic aneurysm repair in symptomatic high-risk patients. J Endovasc Ther. 2006;13(5):681–6.

Chapter 20
Maldeployment of the Contralateral Limb During EVAR

Robert P. Allison, Anna Maria Belli, Joo-Young Chun, Raymond Chung, Raj Das, Andrew England, Karen Flood, Marie-France Giroux, Richard G. McWilliams, Robert Morgan, Nik Papadakos, Jai V. Patel, Raf Patel, Uday Patel, Lakshmi Ratnam, Reddi Prasad Yadavali, and John Rose

Abstract This case illustrates a method of managing the complication of deploying the contralateral limb outside the main body during an EVAR procedure.

Keywords Complications • EVAR • Maldeployed limb

R.P. Allison
Department of Interventional Radiology,
University Hospitals Southampton,
Southampton, Hampshire, UK

A.M. Belli
Department of Radiology,
St. George's Hospital and Medical School,
Blackshaw Road, London SW17 0RE, UK
e-mail: anna.belli@stgeorges.nhs.uk

J.-Y. Chun • R. Chung • R. Das
R. Morgan • N. Papadakos
Department of Radiology,
St. George's Hospital, London, UK

A. England
Department of Radiography,
University of Salford, Manchester, UK

K. Flood
Department of Vascular Radiology,
Leeds General Infirmary, Leeds, UK

M.-F. Giroux
Department of Radiology,
CHUM-Centre Hospitalier de l'Université de Montréal,
Montreal, QC, Canada

R.G. McWilliams
Department of Radiology,
Royal Liverpool University Hospital, Liverpool, UK

J.V. Patel
Department of Radiology,
The Leeds Teaching Hospitals NHS Trust,
Leeds, West Yorkshire, UK

R. Patel
Department of Radiology,
The Leeds Teaching Hospitals NHS Trust,
Leeds, West Yorkshire, UK
e-mail: rafpatel@gmail.com

U. Patel
Department of Diagnostic Radiology,
St. George's Hospital and Medical School,
Blackshaw Road, SW17 0QT London, UK
e-mail: uday.patel@stgeorges.nhs.uk

L. Ratnam
Department of Radiology,
St. George's Hospital,
Blackshaw Road, SW17 0QT London, UK
e-mail: lakshmi.ratnam@nhs.net

R.P. Yadavali
Department of Radiology,
Aberdeen Royal Infirmary, Aberdeen, UK

J. Rose
Department of Interventional Radiology,
Freeman Hospital, Newcastle Upon Tyne Hospitals NHS Trust,
Newcastle upon Tyne, UK

Chapter 20. Maldeployment of the Contralateral Limb

Case History

An 83-year-old man underwent attempted implantation of a bifurcated stent graft for an asymptomatic AAA. The main body of the device was inserted through the right common femoral artery. Following this, the contralateral limb was inadvertently deployed outside the short leg and the proximal portion lay within the aneurysm sac (Fig. 20.1a). As a temporizing maneuver, a right-to-left femorofemoral

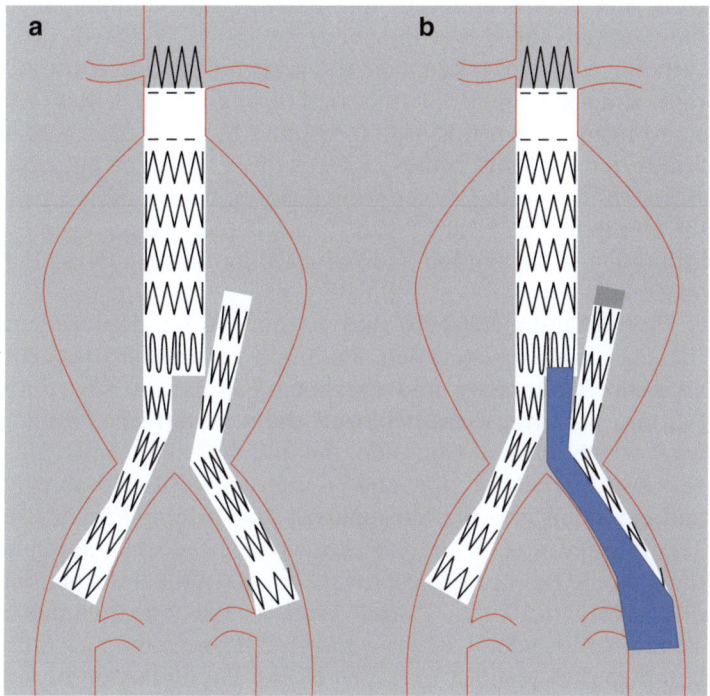

FIGURE 20.1 (a) Diagram demonstrating the position of the initial maldeployed contralateral limb; (b) diagram demonstrating the results from the corrective procedure. The original contralateral limb has been occluded using embolization coils. Blood flow to the left external iliac artery is now provided by an additional limb running alongside the maldeployed component

crossover graft was inserted, and the patient was transferred to a tertiary center for specialist management. A decision was made to establish flow in both iliac limbs and remove the narrow-caliber crossover graft.

Procedure

Preliminary angiography in the operating theater demonstrated that the contralateral gate was still patent. A guidewire was passed alongside the existing left common iliac limb and advanced into the aneurysm sac. A reversed curve catheter was then taken over the graft bifurcation from the right and a hydrophilic wire passed through the left stump. A snare from the left was used to capture this guidewire and a femorofemoral wire achieved. Over this a left-sided catheter was advanced into the suprarenal aorta. Confirmation that the stump had been successfully cannulated was achieved by inflating a Coda balloon (Cook Inc, Bloomington, IN) in the contralateral gate.

Embolization coils (10 and 12 mm) were deployed at the top of the existing left iliac limb in order to prevent an endoleak directly into the aneurysm sac. A new limb (12 mm × 122 mm) was deployed over the left-sided guidewire which passed alongside the old left iliac limb. This was overlapped by one and a quarter stents proximally and extended into the left external iliac artery (Fig. 20.1b). The internal iliac artery was known to be occluded. Since there would be competition for space within the left common iliac artery, a 10 mm Palmaz Genesis balloon-expandable stent (Cordis, Miami, FL) was inserted through the new limb and post-dilated to 12 mm (Fig. 20.2a). The transition of the stent graft into the left external iliac artery was also treated with a 12 mm × 60 mm Wallstent (Boston Scientific, Natick, MA). Post-deployment angiography showed no flow through this segment of vessel; however, embolectomy was performed and flow reestablished. Completion angiography demonstrated good flow down both iliac limbs and no evidence of endoleak. The patient made an uneventful recovery and there were no hemodynamic problems in follow-up.

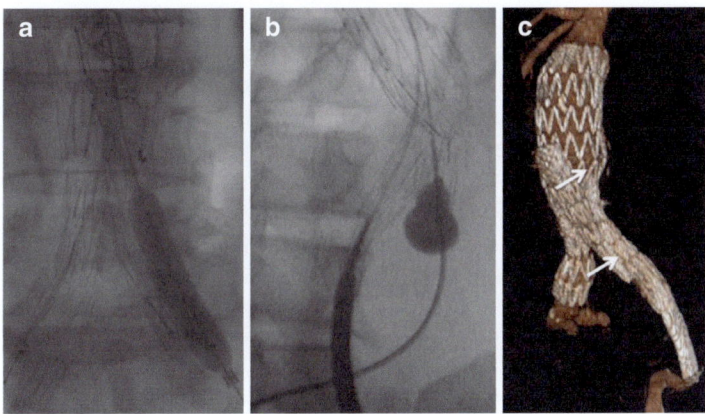

FIGURE 20.2 (**a**) At reintervention, the new iliac limb has been correctly deployed within the short limb of the main body and the external iliac artery on the left side. With the possibility of competition for space, a Palmaz stent has been deployed inside the new limb and is being fully dilated with an angioplasty balloon; (**b**) inflation of a molding balloon to confirm successful cannulation of the main body short limb. The "button-mushroom" appearance of the molding balloon confirms that the guidewire is well positioned through the lumen of the contralateral gate and continues into the main body of the device; (**c**) volume-rendered follow-up CT image demonstrating the position of the deployed stent graft with the "new" iliac limb correctly deployed alongside the maldeployed contralateral limb (*arrows*)

Discussion

Contralateral limb catheterization is one of the critical steps during modular infrarenal EVAR. Both stent-graft design and aneurysm morphology can make cannulation of the contralateral limb problematic. Malpositioning of a contralateral iliac limb can contribute to EVAR failure and may necessitate conversion to open repair. Data from the EUROSTAR registry record that conversion to open surgical repair was required in 2–3 % of patients.

Several methods to ensure that the contralateral guidewire is situated inside the main body of the stent graft have been described. The simplest is to advance a pigtail catheter over a guidewire and reform the catheter in the main body of the device. The catheter is then rotated under fluoroscopy; if the pigtail rotates easily within the confines of the device, then the catheter is within the stent graft. If not, then the catheter may be located between the device and the aneurysm wall. Other options include lateral rotation of the image intensifier while visualizing the guidewire and catheter within the main device body or to inflate a molding balloon such as the Coda balloon in the short limb, and a "button-mushroom" appearance to the Coda balloon will confirm successful cannulation (Fig. 20.2b).

Cannulation can be made easier by appropriate selection of the most suitable access side for the main body; this can be achieved by careful review of a patient's anatomy on preoperative imaging. Knowledge and skill in using a variety of different selective catheters and guidewires is necessary. If access to the main body of the device cannot be achieved directly from the contralateral femoral artery, then passing a guidewire over the aortic bifurcation and snaring it can be performed as in this example. Contralateral limb access can also be obtained by advancing a guidewire from the brachial artery.

If malpositioning occurs, then open surgical conversion is a possibility although this is a complex procedure since the aorta is lined with a fully deployed stent graft. Modification of the original bifurcated device into an aorto-uniiliac (AUI) configuration combined with a contralateral occluder is a more favorable alternative with a femorofemoral crossover graft to maintain perfusion down the contralateral leg. Such a device modification requires availability of the necessary components and leaves both legs supplied via a single stent-graft iliac limb. Here we have presented an endovascular solution, which allows direct lower limb perfusion via its own iliac limb (Fig. 20.2c).

Tips

- Successful deployment of the contralateral limb requires careful evaluation of pre-procedural imaging.
- Several techniques may be performed to ensure that the guidewire and catheter are situated in the main body of the device prior to deployment of the contralateral limb.

- Familiarity with modular stent grafts and their radio-opaque markers is recommended in order to ensure correct positioning.
- Endovascular "bailout" of a maldeployed contralateral limb is achievable and is the preferred option prior to any open surgical solution.

Commentary

The authors describe a clever solution to a problem created by previous malposition of the contralateral left limb outside the contralateral limb (CL) opening in the main body of the aortic endograft.

Clearly, placement of the contralateral limb *outside* the CL opening is a fundamental error of EVAR technique, and efforts should be made to avoid it at all costs. The authors have described the techniques that can be used to avoid malposition of the contralateral limb. In the event that CL maldeployment occurs, the standard solution is conversion of the bifurcated endograft morphology to an aortomonoiliac device morphology either by insertion of a new aortomonoiliac device or a converter (W. Cook, Europe), followed by placement of a femorofemoral crossover graft.

In the case description above, the authors describe a novel additional solution to the complication. Operators should consider this option if they encounter the dreaded complication of contralateral limb malposition outside the CL opening.

Further Reading

Buth J, Laheij RJ. Early complications and endoleaks after endovascular abdominal aortic aneurysm repair: report of a multicentre study. J Vasc Surg. 2000;31(1 Pt 1):134–46.

Cuypers PW, Laheij RJ, Buth J. Which factors increase the risk of conversion to open surgery following endovascular abdominal aortic aneurysm repair? The EUROSTAR collaborators. Eur J Vasc Endovasc Surg. 2000;20(2):183–9.

Dawson DL, Terramani TT, Loberman Z, Lumsden AB, Lin PH. Simple technique to ensure coaxial guidewire positioning for placement of iliac limb of modular aortic endograft. J Interv Cardiol. 2003;16(3):223–6.

# Chapter 21
Branch Endograft Disconnection and Impending Type 3 Endoleak Post-EVAR

Robert P. Allison, Anna Maria Belli, Joo-Young Chun, Raymond Chung, Raj Das, Andrew England, Karen Flood, Marie-France Giroux, Richard G. McWilliams, Robert Morgan, Nik Papadakos, Jai V. Patel, Raf Patel, Uday Patel, Lakshmi Ratnam, Reddi Prasad Yadavali, and John Rose

Abstract This case illustrates the importance of follow-up imaging post-EVAR to detect modular disconnection and describes the management in one such case.

Keywords Complications • EVAR • Modular disconnection Stent

R.P. Allison
Department of Interventional Radiology, University Hospitals Southampton, Southampton, Hampshire, UK

A.M. Belli
Department of Radiology, St. George's Hospital and Medical School, Blackshaw Road, London SW17 0RE, UK
e-mail: anna.belli@stgeorges.nhs.uk

J.-Y. Chun • R. Chung • R. Das
R. Morgan • N. Papadakos
Department of Radiology, St. George's Hospital, London, UK

A. England
Department of Radiography, University of Salford,
Manchester, UK

K. Flood
Department of Vascular Radiology, Leeds General Infirmary,
Leeds, UK

M.-F. Giroux
Department of Radiology, CHUM-Centre Hospitalier de
l'Université de Montréal, Montreal, QC, Canada

R.G. McWilliams
Department of Radiology, Royal Liverpool University Hospital,
Liverpool, UK

J.V. Patel
Department of Radiology, The Leeds Teaching Hospitals NHS
Trust, Leeds, West Yorkshire, UK

R. Patel
Department of Radiology,
The Leeds Teaching Hospitals NHS Trust,
Leeds, West Yorkshire, UK
e-mail: rafpatel@gmail.com

U. Patel
Department of Diagnostic Radiology, St. George's Hospital
and Medical School, Blackshaw Road, SW17 0QT London, UK
e-mail: uday.patel@stgeorges.nhs.uk

L. Ratnam
Department of Radiology, St. George's Hospital, Blackshaw Road,
SW17 0QT London, UK
e-mail: lakshmi.ratnam@nhs.net

R.P. Yadavali
Department of Radiology, Aberdeen Royal Infirmary,
Aberdeen, UK

J. Rose
Department of Interventional Radiology, Freeman Hospital,
Newcastle Upon Tyne Hospitals NHS Trust,
Newcastle upon Tyne, UK

Case History

A 68-year-old man with a type 4 thoracoabdominal aneurysm was referred for elective EVAR using a branched graft. The graft was designed with caudally directed branches for the celiac trunk, SMA, and right renal artery. There was a cranially directed branch for the left renal artery, which arose from the aorta considerably lower than the right and had an upward course. The graft was deployed successfully and all the visceral arteries were connected to the parent endograft with covered stents. Specifically, the left renal artery was accessed and a 5×59 mm Atrium stent (Atrium, Hudson, NH) deployed. The aortic end of this stent was dilated to 7 mm within the 6 mm branch of the endograft.

Both the 1-month and 6-month CT scans were unremarkable with all branches patent and the aneurysm diameter stable. On the 1-year CT scan, all branches were patent, but abdominal radiographs taken at the same time showed that the left renal artery endograft was almost completely dislocated from the left renal artery branch, when compared to the baseline images (Fig. 21.1a, b).

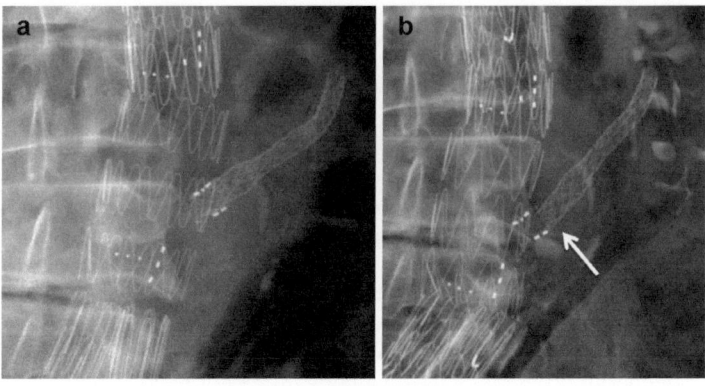

FIGURE 21.1 (**a**) Magnified views (AP) of the left renal artery branch 1 month post branched EVAR showing the baseline position; (**b**) 1-year image demonstrating almost total disconnection (*arrow*) of the left renal stent

Procedure

Preliminary angiography showed almost complete disconnection of the Atrium stent from the upward-pointing left renal branch (Fig. 21.2a), but no visible endoleak. An 8 French sheath was inserted, the branch was accessed, and a Rosen wire (Cook INC, Bloomington, IN) was placed into the left renal artery. A 7 mm × 4 cm Fluency self-expanding stent graft (Bard Peripheral Vascular INC, Tempe, AZ) was placed within the existing renal stent with good overlap into the left renal artery branch on the main aortic endograft (Fig. 21.2b). Completion angiography demonstrated good flow through this segment with no visible complication (Fig. 21.2c). The groin was closed using an 8 French Angio-Seal device (St. Jude Medical, St. Paul, MI). There were no additional complications, and the patient made an uneventful recovery.

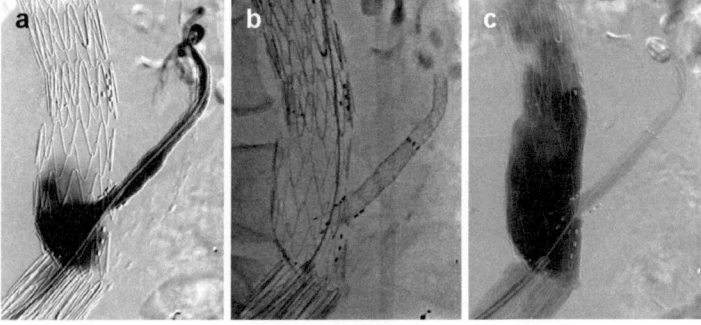

FIGURE 21.2 (**a**) Preliminary angiography showing disconnection of the left renal artery stent with the absence of any related endoleak; (**b**) fluoroscopy image following deployment of a 7 mm × 4 cm Fluency self-expanding stent to bridge the junction between the aortic stent and the original left renal artery stent; (**c**) post-stent angiogram showing the location of the "new" bridging stent which is deliberately extended into the body of the aortic endograft

Discussion

EVAR with a fenestrated or branched endograft offers treatment for patients with challenging anatomy, who are at high risk for open aortic surgery. This technique appears to be feasible and is associated with low mortality. Branched endografts are modular in design. Modularity comes at a price with the modular components having the potential to disconnect during follow-up. For infrarenal endografts this has been reported in around 1 % of patients (Figs. 21.3, 21.4, and 21.5). Branched endografts also have the added possibility that the short endograft that bridges the branch and the target visceral artery may also disconnect from the parent endograft and this presents a new mode of failure. Disconnection results from the component parts being subjected to hemodynamic distraction forces from blood flow. Modular endografts rely solely on frictional forces between overlapping components in order to maintain their structural integrity. Modular disconnection can also result from late anatomical changes during follow-up. Recent advances in dynamic CT imaging have illustrated motion of aortic side branches during the cardiac and respiratory cycles. It has been suggested that this motion may lead to problems at the visceral side branches and may be potentially associated with branch disconnection.

Modular disconnection can be serious and is one of the three possible causes of a type 3 endoleak. Type 3 endoleaks have been associated with aneurysm rupture and therefore warrant prompt reintervention. In most cases the disconnected component remains patent and treatment can be by placing a bridging endograft. Management also focuses on preventative measures both during deployment and in follow-up. Correct component selection and ensuring adequate overlap between components at the time of implantation is essential. Additionally, one of the key objectives of a surveillance

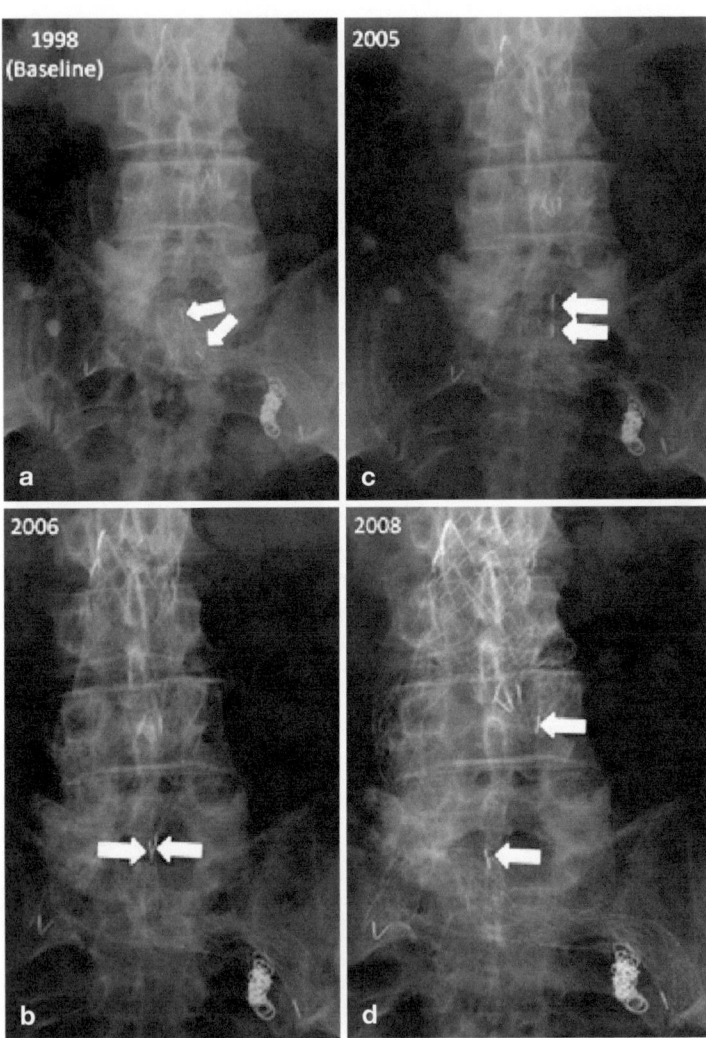

Figure 21.3 (**a, b**) Modular disconnection of a left iliac limb in a Vanguard device. The modular components of the device were overlapping between 1998 and 2005; (**c**) in 2006 there was evidence that there was some component separation; (**d**) by 2008 there was total limb dislocation. *Arrows* indicate the marker positions of the components showing the eventually limb separation

Chapter 21. Branch Endograft Disconnection 163

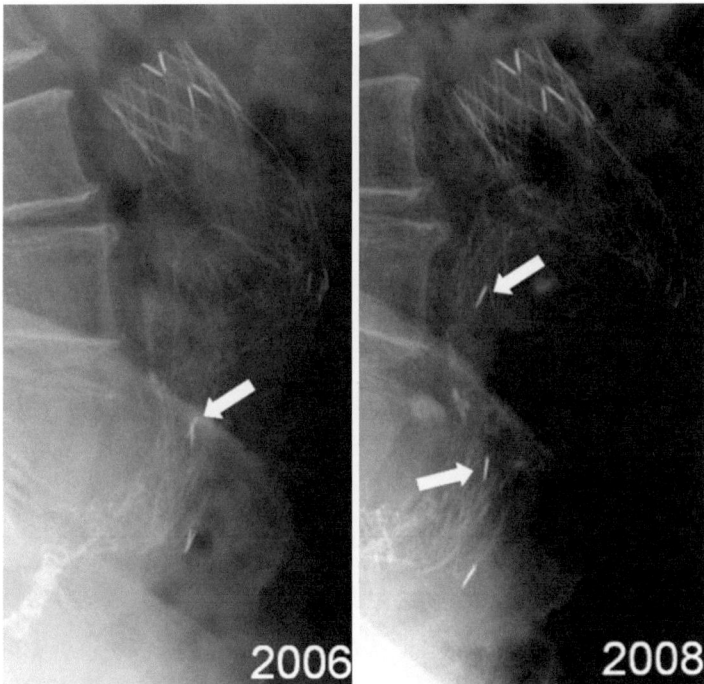

FIGURE 21.4 Same patient as in Fig. 21.3, lateral abdominal radiographs from 2006 to 2008 showing the dislocation of the iliac limb. The proximal component has been pulled up (hose-pipe effect). *Arrows* indicate the marker positions and the movement of the components

program is to review all modular connections and intervene if required before complete disconnection. Dislocations can occur at any time point; Figs. 21.3 and 21.4 show follow-up abdominal radiographs on a patient with a Vanguard stent graft who developed modular disconnection at 10 years from the original implantation. Limb overlap dislocations are less common with latest-generation devices; however, with more complex devices and increased modularity as in multi-branched grafts, there is now the possibility of dislocation at

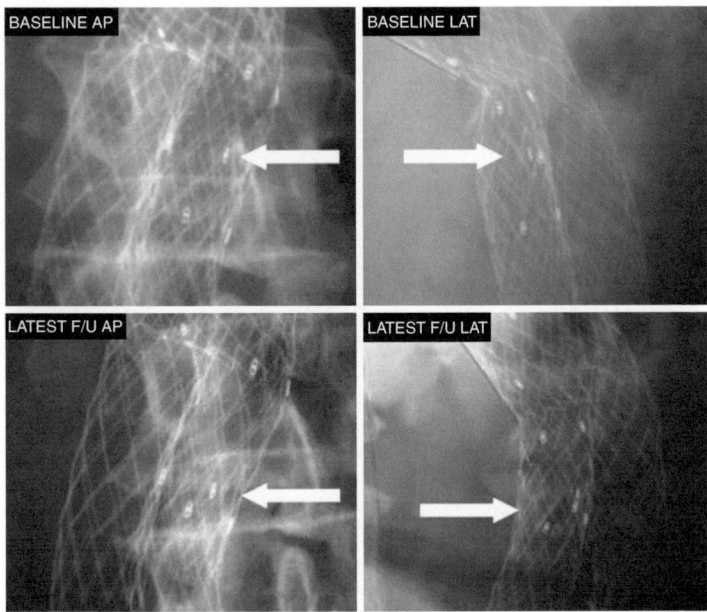

FIGURE 21.5 An AneuRx device (Medtronic, Santa Rosa, CA) with AP and lateral radiographs taken during follow-up. There has been some movement at the modular overlap. This can be identified from serial radiographs and by assessing the changes to the radio-opaque marker positions (*arrows*)

many other sites, which must also be policed during surveillance.

Tips

- Early identification of component separation before dislocation can prevent serious sequelae and allow treatment by an endovascular approach.
- Good understanding of the radio-opaque markers on a stent graft is essential when interpreting follow-up abdominal radiographs. These can often vary between manufacturers and can be an important indicator of impending component dislocation.

Commentary

Dislocation of the bridging endograft between an aortic endograft branch and the target visceral artery is an unusual but reported complication.

Many operators using branched aortic endografts prefer to use self-expanding bridging endografts such as the Fluency device (Bard), as opposed to the less-flexible balloon-expandable endografts as was used in this case. This is because of the perceived, though not proven, increased resistance to endograft separation because a self-expanding endograft may be more tolerant of the constant motion forces that occur during aortic pulsation.

As the authors state, one of the reasons that lifelong imaging follow-up is required in all patients is the detection of modular disconnection, which occurs in a small proportion of patients after conventional, fenestrated, and branched endovascular aneurysm repair. The treatment of modular disconnection is insertion of an additional bridging endograft, which in most cases is not a technically demanding procedure and is associated with high success rates.

Further Reading

Chuter TA. Stent-graft design: the good, the bad and the ugly. Cardiovasc Surg. 2002;10(1):7–13.

Draney MT, Zarins CK, Taylor CA. Three-dimensional analysis of renal artery bending motion during respiration. J Endovasc Ther. 2005;12(3):380–6.

Kaandorp DW, Vasbinder GB, de Haan MW, Kemerink GJ, van Engelshoven JM. Motion of the proximal renal artery during the cardiac cycle. J Magn Reson Imaging. 2000;12(6):924–8.

Muhs BE, Verhoeven EL, Zeebregts CJ, Tielliu IF, Prins TR, Verhagen HJ, et al. Mid-term results of endovascular aneurysm repair with branched and fenestrated endografts. J Vasc Surg. 2006;44(1):9–15.

Powell A, Benenati JF, Becker GJ, Katzen BT, Zemel G, Tummala S. Postoperative management: type I and III endoleaks. Tech Vasc Interv Radiol. 2001;4(4):227–31.

Schlosser FJ, Mojibian HR, Dardik AL, Verhagen HJ, Muhs BE. Pitfalls and complications of fenestrated and branched endografts. Endovascular Today. 2008(February):56–61.

Chapter 22
Hemorrhage Following Percutaneous Nephrostomy

Robert P. Allison, Anna Maria Belli, Joo-Young Chun, Raymond Chung, Raj Das, Andrew England, Karen Flood, Marie-France Giroux, Richard G. McWilliams, Robert Morgan, Nik Papadakos, Jai V. Patel, Raf Patel, Uday Patel, Lakshmi Ratnam, Reddi Prasad Yadavali, and John Rose

Abstract This case discusses the management options for hemorrhage occurring post-nephrostomy insertion with an example from a nephrostomy insertion in an acutely obstructed, septic patient.

Keywords Complications • Nephrostomy • Hemorrhage • Embolization

R.P. Allison
Department of Interventional Radiology, University Hospitals Southampton, Southampton, Hampshire, UK

A.M. Belli
Department of Radiology, St. George's Hospital and Medical School, Blackshaw Road, London SW17 0RE, UK
e-mail: anna.belli@stgeorges.nhs.uk

J.-Y. Chun • R. Chung • R. Das
R. Morgan • N. Papadakos
Department of Radiology, St. George's Hospital, London, UK

A. England
Department of Radiography, University of Salford,
Manchester, UK

K. Flood
Department of Vascular Radiology, Leeds General Infirmary,
Leeds, UK

M.-F. Giroux
Department of Radiology, CHUM-Centre Hospitalier de
l'Université de Montréal, Montreal, QC, Canada

R.G. McWilliams
Department of Radiology, Royal Liverpool University Hospital,
Liverpool, UK

J.V. Patel
Department of Radiology, The Leeds Teaching Hospitals NHS
Trust, Leeds, West Yorkshire, UK

R. Patel
Department of Radiology,
The Leeds Teaching Hospitals NHS Trust,
Leeds, West Yorkshire, UK
e-mail: rafpatel@gmail.com

U. Patel
Department of Diagnostic Radiology, St. George's Hospital
and Medical School, Blackshaw Road, SW17 0QT London, UK
e-mail: uday.patel@stgeorges.nhs.uk

L. Ratnam
Department of Radiology, St. George's Hospital, Blackshaw Road,
SW17 0QT London, UK
e-mail: lakshmi.ratnam@nhs.net

R.P. Yadavali
Department of Radiology, Aberdeen Royal Infirmary,
Aberdeen, UK

J. Rose
Department of Interventional Radiology, Freeman Hospital,
Newcastle Upon Tyne Hospitals NHS Trust,
Newcastle upon Tyne, UK

Case History

A 73-year-old woman presented to interventional radiology with the recent finding of right hydronephrosis and hydroureter. This was evaluated by contrast-enhanced CT of the abdomen and pelvis. Background history included recent appendicectomy. At presentation, the patient was septic with an *E. coli* urinary tract infection and bacteremia. The cause of the hydronephrosis and distal ureteric obstruction was unclear but was suspected to be either secondary to a postinflammatory ureteric stricture following recent pelvic sepsis or related to the finding of bilateral complex ovarian cysts/gynecological pathology.

Procedure

As the patient was septic, urgent right nephrostomy was undertaken. Initial puncture of an upper pole calyx was successfully performed, but guidewire access was difficult and a subsequent fluoroscopic puncture of a posterior interpolar calyx was required. Unfortunately within 6 h of the nephrostomy tube placement, the patient deteriorated with post-procedural bleeding. Urgent arterial phase CT was performed demonstrating that the nephrostomy tube was lying within the renal parenchyma and the right kidney was markedly swollen with multiple areas of contrast extravasation indicating active hemorrhage. A large surrounding retroperitoneal hematoma was present (Fig. 22.1).

Emergency right renal embolization was performed immediately following the CT scan via a 6 French sheath placed in the left common femoral artery; the right renal artery was cannulated using a Cobra C1 catheter. Selective angiograms demonstrated multiple areas of hemorrhage throughout the kidney. Distal selective coils were placed initially; however coils within more proximal renal arterial branches were required to control the hemorrhage.

Subsequently the patient recovered in intensive care with positive-pressure ventilation, hemofiltration, and multiple antibiotic regimens. Surgery was not necessary but subsequent

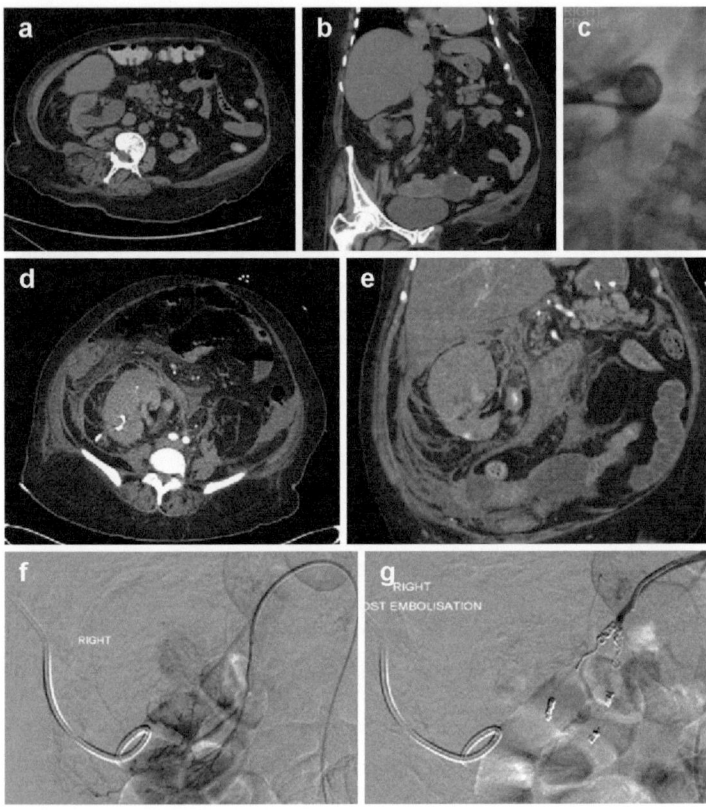

FIGURE 22.1 (**a, b**) are axial and coronal CT images showing a dilated and obstructed right kidney. (**c**) was taken soon after insertion of a nephrostomy catheter under combined ultrasound and fluoroscopic guidance, after failed upper pole access. (**d, e**) are post-contrast CT images showing a large right subcapsular hematoma. (**f, g**) are angiographic images taken before and after embolization. Multiple distal arteriolar bleeding points were seen and these were embolized using micro-coils

drainage of perinephric hematoma was performed. Following recovery, the patient has required dialysis for ongoing chronic renal impairment.

Discussion

Nephrostomy insertion has a major hemorrhagic complication rate of 2–4 %, requiring blood transfusion or re-intervention/embolization. Minor hematuria is seen in almost every case of percutaneous nephrostomy insertion and is usually self-limiting. The technique of accurate puncture is important to prevent hemorrhagic complications with care to traverse the relatively avascular plane of Brödel, which lies between the dorsal and ventral divisions of the renal arteries. In the normal orientation of the kidney, this zone of safety corresponds to the long axes of the posterior-facing calyces.

In most instances, significant bleeding noted at the time of nephrostomy can be controlled by tamponade of the track with a nephrostomy catheter for a small-bore track or with a balloon dilation catheter for large tracts. When this fails or when significant blood loss develops several days after nephrostomy tube placement or removal, angiographic evaluation for identification of a renal arteriovenous fistula, pseudoaneurysm, or vessel laceration is indicated. Most of these vascular injuries can be managed with transcatheter embolization, and surgical intervention is rarely necessary. Selective embolization of the branch artery involved should lead to infarction of only a small segment of kidney, with preservation of functioning renal parenchyma.

In this case, the nephrostomy tube had become displaced and this may have precipitated the perirenal and retroperitoneal hemorrhage, and safe and reliable securing of the nephrostomy tube is an important factor.

Tips

- The safest entry point for nephrostomy insertion is a posterior-facing calyx of the lower pole. In the lower pole the collecting system is consistently the most posterior compared to the arteries or veins. However, in the upper pole the posterior division artery or the upper pole segmental artery lies behind the collecting system (at the level of the renal pelvis or infundibulum), and upper pole punctures are theoretically more likely to injure a vessel.

- The more medial the puncture, the more likely that a large arterial division may be injured. Medial (infundibular or pelvic) upper pole punctures should be especially avoided.
- The Brödel's line describes the watershed zone between the anterior and posterior division arteries and circumvents the periphery of the kidney. Puncture along this line should reduce the risk of major vascular injury.

Commentary

The range and frequency of expected complications after nephrostomy have been thoroughly documented; and extant practice guidelines list the acceptable thresholds for each of these. Hemorrhage is more common in those with a bleeding tendency and in those where the normal safe anatomical principles (discussed above) are not observed. Regarding clotting status, practice guidelines advise that the INR should be <1.5 and the platelet count >50,000. Intuitively, the risk of bleeding should be lower after micro needle access, but this has not been proven.

When it does occur, management should be governed by the clinical impact of the renal hemorrhage. Minor hematuria does not require any specific measures as it will stop in a few days. Slow bleeds with falling blood hemoglobin level should be treated expectantly. These are due to either venous bleeding or a small arterial bleed, and continued catheter drainage will tamponade the bleed until it naturally heals. Once the urine is clear, catheter removal should be performed under controlled conditions in the interventional suite. The catheter should be carefully removed over the guidewire and immediately replaced if bleeding recurs to re-tamponade the track, and angiography and embolization of the bleeding artery undertaken. Angiography may not reveal any active bleeding unless the catheter is removed during contrast injection.

If however the bleed is clinically significant from the start, then immediate angiography and embolization should be performed as in this case. Coils are the preferred embolic agent for post-nephrostomy arterial bleeds.

Further Reading

ACR – SIR – Practice guideline for the performance of percutaneous nephrostomy. http://www.acr.org/~/media/ACR/Documents/PGTS/guidelines/Percutaneous_Nephrostomy.pdf. Accessed 10 Feb 2013.

Clark TW, Abraham RJ, Flemming BK. Is routine micropuncture access necessary for percutaneous nephrostomy? A randomized trial. Can Assoc Radiol J. 2002;53:87–91.

Consensus guidelines for periprocedural management of coagulation status and hemostasis risk in percutaneous image-guided interventions. http://cirse.org/files/File/SOP/Periprocedural.pdf. Accessed 10 Feb 2013.

Dyer RB, Regan JD, Kavanagh PV, Khatod EG, Chen MY, Zagoria RJ. Percutaneous nephrostomy with extensions of the technique: step by step. Radiographics. 2002;22(3):503–25. Review.

Horton A, Ratnam L, Madigan J, Munneke G, Patel U. Nephrostomy – why, how and what to look out for. Imaging. 2008;20:29–37.

Chapter 23
Injury to Bowel Following Transplant Nephrostomy Insertion

Robert P. Allison, Anna Maria Belli, Joo-Young Chun, Raymond Chung, Raj Das, Andrew England, Karen Flood, Marie-France Giroux, Richard G. McWilliams, Robert Morgan, Nik Papadakos, Jai V. Patel, Raf Patel, Uday Patel, Lakshmi Ratnam, Reddi Prasad Yadavali, and John Rose

Abstract This case illustrates the management of bowel perforation during transplant nephrostomy insertion. Tips for reducing the risk of this occurring are discussed.

Keywords Complications • Transplant nephrostomy • Bowel perforation

R.P. Allison
Department of Interventional Radiology, University Hospitals Southampton, Southampton, Hampshire, UK

A.M. Belli
Department of Radiology, St. George's Hospital and Medical School, Blackshaw Road, London SW17 0RE, UK
e-mail: anna.belli@stgeorges.nhs.uk

J.-Y. Chun • R. Chung • R. Das
R. Morgan • N. Papadakos
Department of Radiology, St. George's Hospital, London, UK

A. England
Department of Radiography, University of Salford,
Manchester, UK

K. Flood
Department of Vascular Radiology, Leeds General Infirmary,
Leeds, UK

M.-F. Giroux
Department of Radiology, CHUM-Centre Hospitalier de
l'Université de Montréal, Montreal, QC, Canada

R.G. McWilliams
Department of Radiology, Royal Liverpool University Hospital,
Liverpool, UK

J.V. Patel
Department of Radiology, The Leeds Teaching Hospitals NHS
Trust, Leeds, West Yorkshire, UK

R. Patel
Department of Radiology,
The Leeds Teaching Hospitals NHS Trust,
Leeds, West Yorkshire, UK
e-mail: rafpatel@gmail.com

U. Patel
Department of Diagnostic Radiology, St. George's Hospital
and Medical School, Blackshaw Road, SW17 0QT London, UK
e-mail: uday.patel@stgeorges.nhs.uk

L. Ratnam
Department of Radiology, St. George's Hospital, Blackshaw Road,
SW17 0QT London, UK
e-mail: lakshmi.ratnam@nhs.net

R.P. Yadavali
Department of Radiology, Aberdeen Royal Infirmary,
Aberdeen, UK

J. Rose
Department of Interventional Radiology, Freeman Hospital,
Newcastle Upon Tyne Hospitals NHS Trust,
Newcastle upon Tyne, UK

Case History

A 55-year-old man presented with deterioration in renal function and hydronephrosis of a right renal transplant, 1 week after the removal of a ureteric stent. The transplant surgery had taken place 9 months prior to this presentation with subsequent recurrent episodes of obstruction due to a distal ureteric stricture, which had undergone previous ureteric dilatation and stenting.

Procedure

An ultrasound (US)-guided needle puncture was performed of an interpolar calyx of the transplant kidney. On US, it was noted that the renal capsule was approximately 2 cm below the skin surface with no intervening structures. A Seldinger technique was used to gain access to the collecting system and serial dilatation was performed of the tract. An 8 Fr locking percutaneous nephrostomy tube (PCN) was inserted. A nephrostogram demonstrated tapering of the distal ureter just beyond a number of surgical ligation clips consistent with the known distal ureteric stricture (Fig. 23.1a). There was

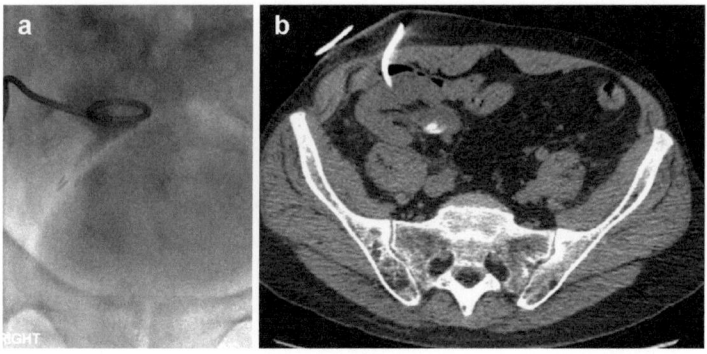

FIGURE 23.1 (a) Post-nephrostomy insertion nephrostogram; (b) on the CT scan, the nephrostomy tubing appears to traverse an overlying small bowel loop before entering the transplant kidney

however contrast drainage into the bladder confirming the presence of a partial obstruction. The nephrostomy tube was secured to the skin using a suture and adhesive dressing.

During the procedure the patient complained of considerable discomfort and in particular of suprapubic abdominal pain following dilatation of the tract. The symptoms persisted and did not resolve with catheterization of the urinary bladder. A repeat US was performed at the end of the procedure which revealed no hematoma or perinephric fluid collection and an urgent CT scan was arranged for further assessment.

The CT scan revealed that the nephrostomy had apparently traversed an overlying small bowel loop before entering the kidney (Fig. 23.1b). The case was discussed with the renal transplant surgery team, and it was agreed that a second nephrostomy should be inserted for drainage (leaving the first one in situ). An exploratory laparotomy was performed to remove the first nephrostomy tube and repair any small bowel perforation if present. This was successfully performed. The patient also later underwent excision of the distal ureteric stricture and ureteric reimplantation. All surgical episodes were uneventful, and the patient made an uncomplicated recovery along with an improvement in biochemical markers of renal function.

Discussion

Visceral injury is seen in <0.5 % of cases after PCN, colonic injury being more common. Factors which may increase the risk of injury to adjacent organs, viscera, and bowel include the number of passes and manipulation required to access the system, the approach used or calyx selected for puncture (e.g., a more lateral approach or intercostal approach), the size of the tract created, anatomical variants (e.g., the ectopic kidney, posteriorly positioned colon), and patients with thinner body habitus (due the paucity of intra-abdominal fat). But all of these suspected risk factors are speculative, as the incidence is too low for any formal studies.

Small bowel injury is even less common but can become clinically evident almost immediate due to pain out of proportion to that expected for the procedure (as suspected in our case). A delayed presentation may manifest with bowel obstruction, paralytic ileus, peritonitis, sepsis, or fluid and electrolyte imbalance. Small bowel injury has been reported to be amenable to conservative management, with bowel rest and parenteral nutrition, similar to the management of an enterocutaneous fistula. Surgery is advocated in cases where spontaneous closure is not likely (e.g., short tract, radiation enteritis, an associated inflammatory process, foreign body in the tract, and distal obstruction).

The general complications encountered with renal transplant nephrostomy should be similar to those described in conventional nephrostomy (e.g., sepsis, hemorrhage, vascular injury). As such we were not able to find any similar reports of bowel injury following renal transplant nephrostomy.

The superficial location of a renal transplant in the traditional iliac fossa location should allow good visualization during the US-guided needle puncture and therefore reduce the potential risk of adjacent visceral injury. However in the immediate postoperative period, soft tissue swelling, edema, and hemorrhage may hinder optimal imaging. In addition, a collapsed segment of small bowel, with a paucity of gas or fluid within it, may not be appreciated on US. Unlike conventional nephrostomy, small bowel is more likely to be adjacent to a renal transplant, and therefore this should be considered when performing a nephrostomy in such cases. Careful inspection by US imaging prior to commencing the procedure should be undertaken, and if there is any doubt, cross-sectional imaging may be valuable to assess for potential adjacent and overlying viscera.

Tips

- Careful US imaging prior to commencing the procedure to identify any potential adjacent visceral structures and to select the safest approach for access.

- Cross-sectional imaging should be considered if US imaging is suboptimal or there is suspicion of visceral structures overlying the kidney.
- Early CT imaging if there is any concern that visceral or bowel injury has occurred during nephrostomy.
- Liaise with the surgical team if small bowel injury is suspected to decide on the most appropriate management plan.

Commentary

The expected performance standards for PCN have been published but the data mostly pertain to the native kidneys. Although there are many published series of transplant nephrostomy, the standards for this subset have not been defined. The authors suggest that these should be similar to native PCN, but there are certain extra risks with a transplant PCN.

Although the transplant kidney is superficial, its orientation can be variable. For example, it may lie horizontally, or the renal pelvis may have rotated anteriorly or even be lateral in orientation. Thus initial ultrasound to establish the anatomy is crucial. Any available CT or MRI images are useful for understanding the anatomy. Secondly, as the authors mention, the peritoneum or even bowel loops may drape anteriorly, and superiorly the caecum may be close to the upper pole of a right-sided transplant. These should be excluded. Even then, and if feasible, entry should be a lateral upper pole calyx. This helps avoid not only any draping peritoneum or bowel but also a lateral orientated pelvis/ureter and the major vessels. This is in contradistinction to the native kidney, where the lower pole calyx is anatomically safest.

Further general noteworthy features about transplant PCN are that the capsule of a transplant kidney may be markedly fibrotic, and dilatation and catheter insertion can be difficult. A stiff guidewire and over dilatation of the track by 1–2 Fr compared to the PCN catheter size help.

When the bowel is injured, a conservative policy is best. Most cases will heal if the track is left for a week to let an enterocutaneous fistula mature. But during this period, adequate drainage of the kidney either by a second PCN or a stent may be required, and these should be left in situ until the urinary obstruction is relieved, or a complex urinary fistula may develop. Also the patient should be closely monitored, and any evidence of peritonitis or bowel obstruction should prompt surgical revision.

Further Reading

Gerspach JM, Bellman GC, Stoller ML, Fugelso P. Conservative management of colon injury following percutaneous renal surgery. Urology. 1997;49(6):831–6.

Mostafa SA, Abbaszadeh S, Taheri S, Nourbala MH. Percutaneous nephrostomy for treatment of posttransplant ureteral obstructions. Urol J. 2008;5(2):79–83.

Ramchandani P, Cardella JF, Grassi CJ, Roberts AC, Sacks D, Schwartzberg MS, Lewis CA. Society of Interventional Radiology Standards of Practice Committee. Quality improvement guidelines for percutaneous nephrostomy. J Vasc Interv Radiol. 2003;14(9 Pt 2):S277–81.

Santiago L, Bellman GC, Murphy J, Tan L. Small bowel and splenic injury during percutaneous renal surgery. J Urol. 1998;159(6):2071–2; discussion 2072–3.

Winer AG, Hyams ES, Shah O. Small bowel injury during percutaneous nephrostomy tube placement causing small bowel obstruction. Can J Urol. 2009;16(6):4950–2.

Chapter 24
Renal Arterial Hemorrhage Following Renal Artery Stenting

Robert P. Allison, Anna Maria Belli, Joo-Young Chun, Raymond Chung, Raj Das, Andrew England, Karen Flood, Marie-France Giroux, Richard G. McWilliams, Robert Morgan, Nik Papadakos, Jai V. Patel, Raf Patel, Uday Patel, Lakshmi Ratnam, Reddi Prasad Yadavali, and John Rose

Abstract This case describes hemorrhage following renal artery stenting in which selective embolization was not possible. The main renal artery was coiled to stop the hemorrhage and save the patient.

Keywords Renal artery stent • Complication • Hemorrhage • Embolization

R.P. Allison
Department of Interventional Radiology, University Hospitals Southampton, Southampton, Hampshire, UK

A.M. Belli
Department of Radiology, St. George's Hospital and Medical School, Blackshaw Road, London SW17 0RE, UK
e-mail: anna.belli@stgeorges.nhs.uk

J.-Y. Chun • R. Chung • R. Das
R. Morgan • N. Papadakos
Department of Radiology, St. George's Hospital, London, UK

A. England
Department of Radiography, University of Salford,
Manchester, UK

K. Flood
Department of Vascular Radiology, Leeds General Infirmary,
Leeds, UK

M.-F. Giroux
Department of Radiology, CHUM-Centre Hospitalier de
l'Université de Montréal, Montreal, QC, Canada

R.G. McWilliams
Department of Radiology, Royal Liverpool University Hospital,
Liverpool, UK

J.V. Patel
Department of Radiology, The Leeds Teaching Hospitals NHS
Trust, Leeds, West Yorkshire, UK

R. Patel
Department of Radiology,
The Leeds Teaching Hospitals NHS Trust,
Leeds, West Yorkshire, UK
e-mail: rafpatel@gmail.com

U. Patel
Department of Diagnostic Radiology, St. George's Hospital
and Medical School, Blackshaw Road, SW17 0QT London, UK
e-mail: uday.patel@stgeorges.nhs.uk

L. Ratnam
Department of Radiology, St. George's Hospital,
Blackshaw Road, SW17 0QT London, UK
e-mail: lakshmi.ratnam@nhs.net

R.P. Yadavali
Department of Radiology, Aberdeen Royal Infirmary,
Aberdeen, UK

J. Rose
Department of Interventional Radiology, Freeman Hospital,
Newcastle Upon Tyne Hospitals NHS Trust,
Newcastle upon Tyne, UK

Case History

A 77-year-old gentleman was admitted for elective left renal artery stenting for severe left renal artery stenosis. Previous medical history included atrial fibrillation and chronic renal impairment. Stenting was requested urgently as an inpatient as the patient was suffering with deteriorating renal function and ongoing pulmonary edema.

Preprocedural investigations included CT angiography demonstrating single bilateral renal arteries. The left kidney was of normal size but with a tight stenosis at the origin of the left renal artery. The right kidney was small and also demonstrated a renal artery stenosis.

Procedure

Initial attempts to cannulate the left renal artery were unsuccessful from the left groin; therefore bilateral femoral punctures were performed with 6 Fr arterial sheaths. Five thousand units of heparin were administered. The left renal artery was pre-dilated to 4 mm and a 6×20 mm metallic stent was painlessly deployed, with satisfactory appearances and without any immediate complications (Fig. 24.1).

The patient deteriorated 10 h later and became hemodynamically unstable with abdominal distension. CT abdomen with pre-contrast and arterial phases was performed, demonstrating a large perirenal hematoma with active extravasation of contrast from the upper pole of the left kidney in arterial phase.

Immediate repeat angiography with recannulation of the left renal artery was performed. Angiography demonstrated acute hemorrhage from a small branch in the upper pole of the left kidney. This arterial branch had not been catheterized during the renal stenting procedure therefore the etiology of the hemorrhage was not thought to be guidewire trauma or

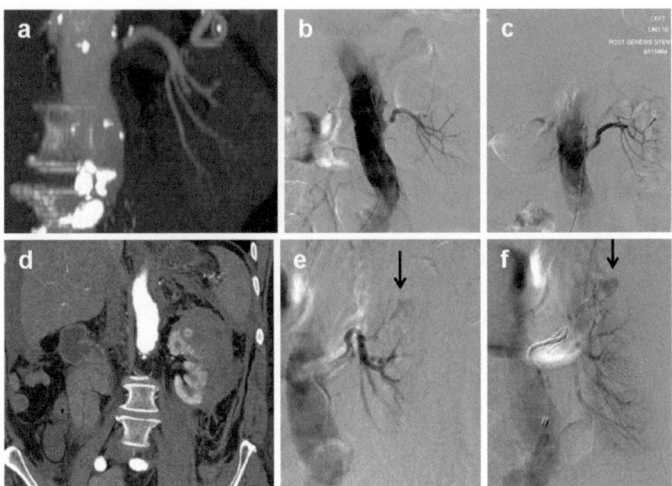

Figure 24.1 (**a**) is a coronal CT image showing left renal artery stenosis, confirmed on catheter angiography (**b**) and that was stented without immediate complication as shown in (**c**). (**d**) is a CT scan undertaken 10 h post-stenting showing a large pericapsular hematoma. Bleeding around the stent was suspected, but on angiography the bleeding was seen to emanate from a peripheral arterial branch (**e, f** *arrows*)

trauma directly from the stent placement. Multiple attempts were made to cannulate the branch feeding the arterial hemorrhage; however this proved difficult due to the tortuosity of the main renal artery and oblique origin of the upper pole branch.

In view of the life-threatening situation, the main renal artery was embolized with multiple coils. Final angiography demonstrated cessation of flow into the left kidney with no evidence of residual active hemorrhage.

Discussion

Hemorrhage shortly after renal stenting is a described complication but is rare. Renal artery stenting is a safe procedure with a low complication rate. Previous studies documenting iatrogenic renal artery injuries occurring after renal artery angioplasty and stenting describe access site hematomas and pseudoaneurysms, contrast-related nephropathy, distal embolization, renal artery rupture, renal artery dissection, and renal artery thrombosis with an overall complication rate of 4.2 % per renal artery and 6.1 % per patient treated.

In this case, as the point of hemorrhage occurred from a small branch in the upper pole of the left kidney, it seems likely that the etiology of the hemorrhage was due to reperfusion. The exact pathophysiological mechanisms are uncertain but have been described as transient hyperperfusion of renal tissue after recanalization of the main renal arterial lumen after percutaneous intervention.

The theory of normal perfusion pressure breakthrough was described by Spetzler et al. in the cerebral circulation and following carotid artery stenting. The mechanism of hyperperfusion in the renal artery is thought to relate to persistent renal artery occlusive disease and hypoperfusion causing compensatory renal artery branch dilation and loss of autoregulation. After revascularization there is resultant hyperperfusion from increased pressure into the distal renal bed which has lost normal autoregulation. An abnormal, hyperperfused renal artery branch vessel might rupture with resultant hemorrhage.

Risk factors for hemorrhage after renal artery stent placement include advanced age (>60 years), high-grade stenosis with poor collateral flow, evidence of chronic ipsilateral hypoperfusion, pre- and postoperative hypertension, diabetes mellitus, generalized arteriosclerosis, coronary artery disease, obesity, small kidney and perioperative anticoagulation, or antiplatelet therapy. Hyperperfusion following stenting may be difficult to predict; however strict control of blood pressure in the periprocedural and immediate post-procedural period may be beneficial, if analogous to the carotid and cerebral circulation.

Post-procedural hemorrhage after renal artery stenting may be less extensive than in this case, and capsular arteries are prone to rupture if exposed to sudden rise in systemic blood pressure. Minor subcapsular hemorrhage or hematoma without hemodynamic instability may be successfully treated by conservative measures with the option of transcatheter embolization if required. In this case, the patient's hemodynamic instability and tortuosity of the renal artery meant that superselective embolization was not possible and the main renal artery required coiling, which was successfully performed.

Tips

- Hemodynamic instability soon after an interventional procedure heralds a major complication, usually bleeding; but other causes such as septicemia and an unrelated cardiac event should also be considered.
- Immediate arterial phase CT scanning should be undertaken.
- If CT scan cannot be performed, then urgent catheter angiography should be considered.
- Embolization should always be as selective as possible. But if not feasible, then proximal embolization should be undertaken. Organ loss is better than losing the patient.

Commentary

Generically speaking, bleeding is the most common and when severe, the most worrying complication after any interventional procedure. There are some predictable risk factors, and these should be sought for and controlled, e.g., clotting status. Each procedure also has its own high-risk technical factors, e.g., a high femoral artery puncture or a medial renal or hepatic puncture during nephrostomy or biliary drainage, respectively, and these should also be sought and controlled for. Regarding angioplasty and arterial stenting, careful sizing of the artery and balloon/stent choice are important. During dilatation the inflation pressure limits for the particular device should not be exceeded, as balloon rupture can tear the artery.

However, rarely the organ or artery may bleed for undefinable reasons. As the images show, the bleeding point was from a distal artery, well away from the site of the stenting. There are cases of guidewire perforation leading to arterial injury, but this was not the case here. The authors have suggested hyperperfusion as the explanation, and whereas this can only remain a hypothesis, the case describes how the interventionalist should be prepared to undertake a less selective embolization if the situation demands. Another rare situation when more extensive renal bleeding may be seen is when a large subcapsular hematoma collects. This can strip the capsule leaving a raw oozing renal surface due to rupture of the capsular arteries. On angiography, multiple distal bleeding points will be seen and again complete renal embolization is necessary.

An additional learning point from this case is the importance of proper patient counselling when consent is obtained for any interventional procedure. Organ loss as a result of an interventional complication is a rare event, but the possibility should always be considered.

Further Reading

Axelrod DJ, Freeman H, Pukin L, Guller J, Mitty HA. Guide wire perforation leading to fatal perirenal hemorrhage from transcortical collaterals after renal artery stent placement. J Vasc Interv Radiol. 2004;15(9):985–7.

Kang KP, Lee S, Kim W, Han YM. Renal subcapsular hematoma: a consequence of reperfusion injury of long standing renal artery stenosis. Electrol Blood Press. 2007;5:136–9.

Morris CS, Bonnevie GJ, Najarian KE. Nonsurgical treatment of acute iatrogenic renal artery injuries occurring after renal artery angioplasty and stenting. AJR Am J Roentgenol. 2001;177(6):1353–7.

Spetzler RF, Wilson CB, Weinstein P, Mehdorn M, Townsend J, Telles D. Normal perfusion pressure breakthrough theory. Clin Neurosurg. 1978;25:651–72.

Xia D, Chen SW, Zhang HK, Wang S. Renal subcapsular haematoma: an unusual complication of renal artery stenting. Chin Med J (Engl). 2011;124(9):1438–40.

Chapter 25
Pyrexia After Tumor Embolization: Infection Versus Post-embolization Syndrome

Robert P. Allison, Anna Maria Belli, Joo-Young Chun, Raymond Chung, Raj Das, Andrew England, Karen Flood, Marie-France Giroux, Richard G. McWilliams, Robert Morgan, Nik Papadakos, Jai V. Patel, Raf Patel, Uday Patel, Lakshmi Ratnam, Reddi Prasad Yadavali, and John Rose

Abstract This case describes the development and treatment of an abscess following embolization of a neuroendocrine tumor metastasis within the liver. The features of abscess formation and post-embolization syndrome are discussed along with treatment strategies.

Keywords Embolization • Complications • Post-embolization syndrome • Abscess

---

R.P. Allison
Department of Interventional Radiology,
University Hospitals Southampton, Southampton, Hampshire, UK

A.M. Belli
Department of Radiology, St. George's Hospital and Medical School, Blackshaw Road, London SW17 0RE, UK
e-mail: anna.belli@stgeorges.nhs.uk

J.-Y. Chun • R. Chung • R. Das
R. Morgan • N. Papadakos
Department of Radiology, St. George's Hospital, London, UK

A. England
Department of Radiography, University of Salford,
Manchester, UK

K. Flood
Department of Vascular Radiology, Leeds General Infirmary,
Leeds, UK

M.-F. Giroux
Department of Radiology, CHUM-Centre Hospitalier de
l'Université de Montréal, Montreal, QC, Canada

R.G. McWilliams
Department of Radiology, Royal Liverpool University Hospital,
Liverpool, UK

J.V. Patel
Department of Radiology, The Leeds Teaching Hospitals NHS
Trust, Leeds, West Yorkshire, UK

R. Patel
Department of Radiology,
The Leeds Teaching Hospitals NHS Trust,
Leeds, West Yorkshire, UK
e-mail: rafpatel@gmail.com

U. Patel
Department of Diagnostic Radiology, St. George's Hospital
and Medical School, Blackshaw Road, SW17 0QT London, UK
e-mail: uday.patel@stgeorges.nhs.uk

L. Ratnam
Department of Radiology, St. George's Hospital, Blackshaw Road,
SW17 0QT London, UK
e-mail: lakshmi.ratnam@nhs.net

R.P. Yadavali
Department of Radiology, Aberdeen Royal Infirmary,
Aberdeen, UK

J. Rose
Department of Interventional Radiology, Freeman Hospital,
Newcastle Upon Tyne Hospitals NHS Trust,
Newcastle upon Tyne, UK

Case History

A 65-year-old gentleman with a known neuroendocrine tumor (NET) was referred to the IR department for embolization of widespread hepatic metastases. The indication was control of tumor bulk rather than palliation of the symptoms of carcinoid syndrome.

Procedure

Following a right common femoral artery puncture and placement of a 5 Fr vascular sheath, the common hepatic artery was accessed via the coeliac trunk. Angiography demonstrated a very large right-sided hypervascular liver mass. The right hepatic artery was superselected with a 2.7 Fr microcatheter, and the tumor was embolized with 100–300 µm size Contour PVA particles. Completion angiography demonstrated significant arterial devascularization of the right-sided liver segments with continued perfusion of the left lobe and a patent right and left portal vein.

The patient remained in hospital for just over a week post-treatment due to prolonged symptoms of post-embolization syndrome. The CT scan before discharge (not shown) demonstrated local cavitation and tumor necrosis. He then re-presented 5 weeks later due to lethargy, worsening but vague abdominal pain and fevers.

Initial CXR (Fig. 25.1a) and subsequent unenhanced CT (Fig. 25.1b) demonstrated an enormous air-containing cavity within the liver (with an air-fluid level and classical "soap bubble" appearance). Given the patient's clinical presentation and raised inflammatory markers, this was consistent with a hepatic abscess.

Views on US were somewhat hampered by the large amount of gas within the cavity, but a 12 Fr pigtail drain was inserted without complication, via an intercostal approach, into the cavity with rapid drainage of purulent fluid. The drain remained secure in the abscess cavity for 8 weeks with the progress of the residual collection followed by interval USS.

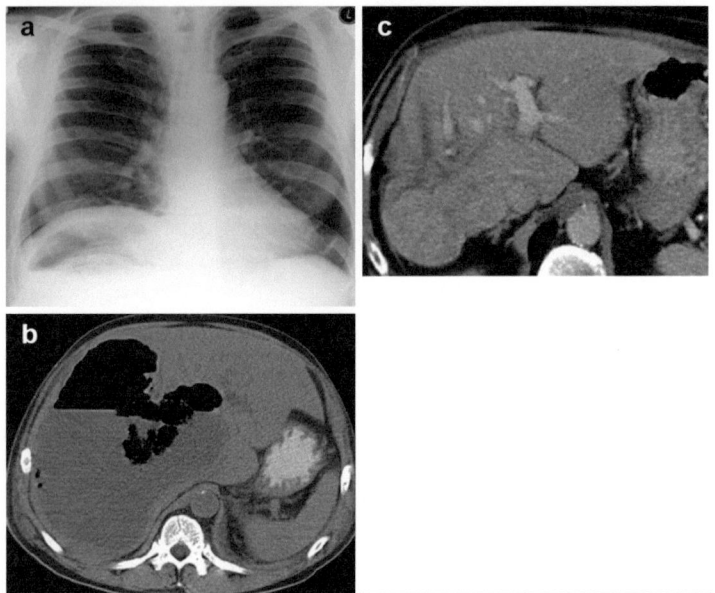

FIGURE 25.1 (**a**) CXR 6 weeks post-embolization; (**b**) unenhanced CT 6 weeks post-embolization; (**c**) CT 3 months following drain placement

With only a small residual collection and no further output, the drain was removed and the patient discharged well. CT scan at 3 months demonstrated a shrunken right hepatic lobe and a reduction in volume of the liver metastases (Fig. 25.1c). The patient remained asymptomatic at this stage.

However, by the time of a 5 month follow up CT, the metastasis had progressed and the patient succumbed to his disease a few months later.

Discussion

The reported incidence of pyogenic abscess formation following hepatic artery embolization is in the region of 1 %, and the risk is generally increased by the presence of a biliary stent or a previous biliary bypass. Significant liver abscess formation requiring percutaneous drainage, as in this case, is extremely rare after embolization of NET metastases providing that the embolization is limited. When embolizing NET liver metastases, a semi-selective catheter position is appropriate so that several tumor nodules in 1–2 liver segments are treated. However, in general, no more than one-third of the liver volume should be embolized in order to reduce the risk of severe post-embolization syndrome and/or abscess formation. As with particulate embolization of any lesion, in any organ one should proceed with caution and cease when there is reduction in the forward flow of contrast. It is good practice to record the initial position of the microcatheter tip with a short DSA run prior to starting the embolization and to perform further "check" interval angiograms during extensive embolization to monitor progress.

In this case a large volume of PVA was steadily injected into the right hepatic artery nonselectively over a short time period. Fortunately the completion angiogram showed that although the right hepatic territory was completely devascularized, the left hepatic artery was patent and there was normal portal venous flow into the liver. There was no evidence of extrahepatic embolization.

The use of small embolic particles (100–300 μm) is thought to allow better penetration of the center of liver metastases and should produce more consistent tumor necrosis, an important factor when trying to gain control of an indolent neoplasm such as NET. However, the use of smaller particles (<300 μm), particularly when used nonselectively as in this case, should be balanced against the increased risk of infarcting non-tumor liver and damaging the blood supply to the biliary tree. Where a large volume of "non-tumor" liver has been inadvertently embolized, it is usually wise to give an appropriate prophylactic antibiotic.

Tips

- Overzealous hepatic artery embolization can lead to significant ischemia. To minimize this when treating large lesions, both patience and repeated check angiography are recommended.

- Tumor necrosis can be expected following embolization and can appear similar to an abscess on CT; differentiation is on clinical grounds.
- US-guided drainage is often straightforward but gas within a cavity can limit views. Although not needed in this case, CT guidance may be necessary.
- Drains for a large abscess will often need to be in for a considerable amount of time, and adequate fixation to the skin is essential.
- Abscesses result from biliary sepsis/ischemia due to the reliance of the biliary system on supply from the hepatic artery, unlike the liver parenchyma which has a dual supply.

Commentary

The post-embolization syndrome (PES) is an enigmatic but common event, and its main features are nausea, mild spikes of temperature, and pain around the embolization site. The exact cause is unknown. Blood parameters are elevated with raised C reactive protein, ESR, and white blood cell count. All these features are of course similar to infection and present an immediate clinical conundrum – is this just post-embolization syndrome or is there an infection as well? Typically, PES will begin to improve after 48 h, and the nausea and pain will abate although minor fever (usually around the 37.5 °C mark) may continue for up to 4–5 days.

Abscess after embolization is seen in 0.3–4.8 % of cases, depending on tumor/organ type. As the authors observe, imaging may not help. The infarcted volume will develop gas (nitrogen released by infarcted tissue) within 1–2 days and may even show a degree of peripheral or rim enhancement and thus be indistinguishable from an abscess. Initially this clinical scenario is best treated expectantly with antipyretics and antiemetics. Blood cultures should be sent, but antibiotics not commenced unless there is compelling evidence of a superadded infection. If the patient's clinical state (symptoms and acute phase markers) continues to worsen, then an abscess should be suspected. In which case, drainage possibly with a large-bore catheter is usually necessary.

It is not proven whether prophylactic antibiotics may reduce the risk of abscess formation, but these can be given during the embolization process. The impact of the PES may be suppressed with a short course of corticosteroids but this is not routine policy. The use of other anti-inflammatory agents (e.g., NSAIDs) to suppress the PES has not been formally evaluated, but anecdotally they are of value.

Further Reading

Angle JF, Siddiqi NH, Wallace MJ, Kundu S, Stokes LA, Wojak JC, Cardella JF. Quality improvement guidelines for percutaneous transcatheter embolization. J Vasc Interv Radiol. 2010;21:1479–86.

Bissler JJ, Recadio J, Donnelly LF, Johnson ND. Reduction of postembolization syndrome after ablation of renal angiomyolipoma. Am J Kidney Dis. 2002;39(5):966–71.

Mezhir J, Fong Y, et al. Pyogenic abscess after hepatic artery embolisation: a rare but potentially lethal complication. J Vasc Interv Radiol. 2011;22:177–82.

Stewart MJ, Warbey VS, et al. Neuroendocrine tumours: role of interventional radiology in therapy. Radiographics. 2008;28:1131–45.

Chapter 26
Arterioportal Fistula and Liver Hemorrhage After Radiofrequency Ablation and TACE

Robert P. Allison, Anna Maria Belli, Joo-Young Chun, Raymond Chung, Raj Das, Andrew England, Karen Flood, Marie-France Giroux, Richard G. McWilliams, Robert Morgan, Nik Papadakos, Jai V. Patel, Raf Patel, Uday Patel, Lakshmi Ratnam, Reddi Prasad Yadavali, and John Rose

Abstract This case demonstrates development and treatment of an arterioportal fistula following radiofrequency ablation (RFA). The patient underwent combined procedure of RFA followed by transarterial chemoembolization. At angiography the fistula was visualized and treated with coil embolization.

Keywords Radiofrequency ablation • Transarterial chemoembolization • Complication • Arterioportal fistula

---

R.P. Allison
Department of Interventional Radiology,
University Hospitals Southampton,
Southampton, Hampshire, UK

A.M. Belli
Department of Radiology, St. George's Hospital and Medical School, Blackshaw Road,
London SW17 0RE, UK
e-mail: anna.belli@stgeorges.nhs.uk

J.-Y. Chun • R. Chung
R. Das • R. Morgan • N. Papadakos
Department of Radiology, St. George's Hospital, London, UK

A. England
Department of Radiography, University of Salford, Manchester, UK

K. Flood
Department of Vascular Radiology,
Leeds General Infirmary, Leeds, UK

M.-F. Giroux
Department of Radiology, CHUM-Centre Hospitalier
de l'Université de Montréal, Montreal, QC, Canada

R.G. McWilliams
Department of Radiology, Royal Liverpool
University Hospital, Liverpool, UK

J.V. Patel
Department of Radiology,
The Leeds Teaching Hospitals NHS Trust,
Leeds, West Yorkshire, UK

R. Patel
Department of Radiology,
The Leeds Teaching Hospitals NHS Trust,
Leeds, West Yorkshire, UK
e-mail: rafpatel@gmail.com

U. Patel
Department of Diagnostic Radiology,
St. George's Hospital and Medical School,
Blackshaw Road, SW17 0QT London, UK
e-mail: uday.patel@stgeorges.nhs.uk

L. Ratnam
Department of Radiology, St. George's Hospital,
Blackshaw Road, SW17 0QT London, UK
e-mail: lakshmi.ratnam@nhs.net

R.P. Yadavali
Department of Radiology, Aberdeen Royal
Infirmary, Aberdeen, UK

J. Rose
Department of Interventional Radiology,
Freeman Hospital, Newcastle Upon Tyne
Hospitals NHS Trust, Newcastle upon Tyne, UK

Chapter 26. Arterioportal Fistula and Liver Hemorrhage 201

Case History

A 68-year-old gentleman with nonalcoholic steatohepatitis (NASH) cirrhosis and solitary, presumed hepatocellular carcinoma (HCC) attended for an elective combined radiofrequency ablation (RFA) and transarterial chemoembolization (TACE). Pre-procedural contrast-enhanced CT demonstrated the hypervascular lesion/HCC in the right hepatic lobe.

Procedure

Using a standard right common femoral artery approach and a 5 Fr sheath, the common hepatic artery was accessed via the coeliac trunk using a 4 Fr SIM2 catheter. Catheter angiography of the coeliac axis confirmed a hypervascular lesion in the superior aspect of the right hepatic lobe (segment 7), consistent with the 3.5 cm lesion seen on cross-sectional imaging. A 2.7 Fr microcatheter was advanced into the ascending branch of the right hepatic artery and left in place following confirmatory super-selective angiography.

Under ultrasound guidance, a 14 G RFA needle was advanced through the right intercostal route into the tumor in the superior aspect of the right hepatic lobe. The ablation was completed over a period of approximately 15 min; the tines of the RFA probe were then retracted and tract ablation performed during needle withdrawal.

Further angiography via the microcatheter in the superior right hepatic artery demonstrated both some persistence of hypervascularity in the area of the known lesion but also active contrast extravasation along the track of the RFA. Given the small volume of contrast extravasation along the track and hemodynamic stability, we elected to proceed with the TACE. A total of 75 mg of doxorubicin, bound to 100–300 μm drug-eluting beads, was injected in small aliquots. Completion angiography demonstrated a satisfactory reduction in vascularity of the lesion and abolition of the extracapsular bleeding, but an arterioportal venous fistula was

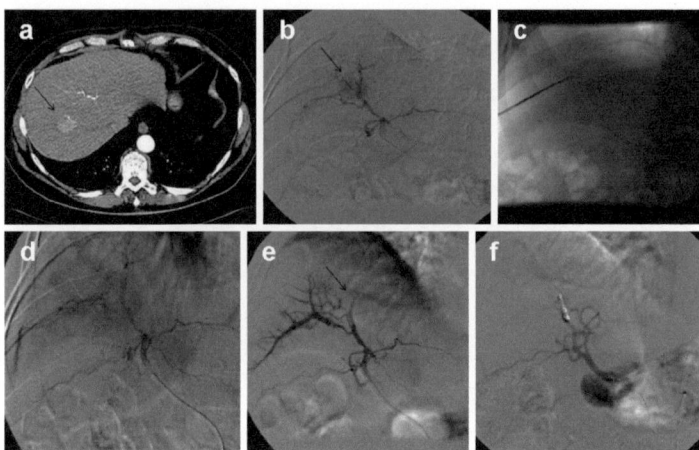

FIGURE 26.1 (**a**) shows an enhancing tumor in the right liver lobe (*arrow*), and this is confirmed as hypervascular (*arrow*) on catheter angiography (**b**). Combined radiofrequency ablation (RFA) and transarterial chemoembolization (TACE) were undertaken. RFA was first undertaken (**c**). The post-RFA angiogram shows a small capsular leak along the RFA tract (**d**). This was felt to be not significant. TACE was undertaken and on the post-TACE angiogram, an arterioportal fistula was seen (*arrow*, **e**). This was embolized with micro-coils (**f**)

revealed on the lateral aspect of the ablated area between the second-order branches of the artery and portal venules. This lesion did not cause any significant immediate clinical problem but was clearly another complication of the RFA. It was considered that there was a small risk of delayed pseudoaneurysm formation and/or bleeding into the post-ablation lesion. Therefore, the fistula was embolized with four platinum coils via the microcatheter. Completion angiography demonstrated barely any flow in the feeding segmental artery and virtually no flow into the fistula. Enhanced CT at both

4 weeks and 3 months did not demonstrate any evidence of residual HCC in the treated segment or new disease.

Discussion

Complications during or following percutaneous RF ablation for liver tumor are very rare and are usually related to the target lesion being very close to major structures in the liver hilum or to adjacent bowel. There is a small reported incidence of biliary sepsis, particularly when ablation is performed in the presence of a biliary enteric bypass. Hemorrhage is very rare where tract ablation is used and tumor seeding along the tract occurs in <1 %. The most dangerous complications are undoubtedly those due to thermal damage to the gallbladder, stomach, or colon when care is not taken to leave a safety margin of at least 1 cm between edges of the adjacent organ and the thermal target volume. The technique of image-guided percutaneous fluid dissection between the target and adjacent hollow organ is described and reduces the potential for such complications.

In this case, despite the use of tract ablation, there was a small leak of blood and contrast along the ablation tract within minutes of the RITA probe being withdrawn. Had this procedure not been planned as a combined treatment, then angiography would not have been performed and the small leak would probably not have come to light. The opening of the arterioportal fistula following the TACE presumably reflects changes in hemodynamics as a result of the occlusion of small arteries feeding the target area. Certainly such fistulae are described both following any transhepatic procedure and as incidental findings in chronic liver disease. AV fistulae are thought to be associated with a small risk of hemorrhage, and it was a simple matter to perform additional coil embolization following the TACE.

Tips

- Tract ablation is very effective in preventing hemorrhage but be aware that it will fail occasionally.
- US scanning of the liver at the end of the procedure can detect subcapsular and peri-hepatic bleeding/fluid, or as demonstrated here it can be seen on angiography.
- A low threshold is reasonable in the treatment of hepatic bleeding even in minor cases.
- Coil embolization was necessary in this case but this will prevent re-treatment by TACE in the same territory.

Commentary

When a complication is seen after an interventional procedure, the operator has the burden of deciding to either leave it alone or embark on active correction. If the complication is immediately symptomatic, then the decision is easy and treatment is necessary. When the complication is subtle or early, then the operator has only his or her judgment and experience at hand. One can only suggest that any active maneuver chosen should be safe and straightforward. In this case the catheter was already in a super-selective position and the embolization was undertaken without any added risk to the patient.

Further Reading

Choi D, Lim H, et al. Liver abscesses after percutaneous radiofrequency ablation for hepatocellular carcinomas: frequency and risk factors. AJR Am J Roentgenol. 2005;184:1860–7.

Ginat D, Saad W. Bowel displacement and protection techniques during percutaneous renal tumour thermal ablation. Tech Vasc Interv Radiol. 2010;13:66–74.

Park HS, Lee SH, et al. Post biopsy arterioportal fistula in patients with hepatocellular carcinoma: clinical significance in transarterial chemoembolisation. AJR Am J Roentgenol. 2006;186:556–61.

Chapter 27
Protrusion of Vena Cava Filter into the Aorta

Robert P. Allison, Anna Maria Belli, Joo-Young Chun, Raymond Chung, Raj Das, Andrew England, Karen Flood, Marie-France Giroux, Richard G. McWilliams, Robert Morgan, Nik Papadakos, Jai V. Patel, Raf Patel, Uday Patel, Lakshmi Ratnam, Reddi Prasad Yadavali, and John Rose

Abstract This case discusses various methods which can be used in attempted retrieval of an IVC filter where the distal hooks of the filter have become incorporated into the caval wall.

Keywords IVC filter retrieval • Complications • Embedded • Incorporated

R.P. Allison
Department of Interventional Radiology,
University Hospitals Southampton,
Southampton, Hampshire, UK

A.M. Belli
Department of Radiology, St. George's Hospital and Medical School, Blackshaw Road,
London SW17 0RE, UK
e-mail: anna.belli@stgeorges.nhs.uk

J.-Y. Chun • R. Chung • R. Das • R. Morgan • N. Papadakos
Department of Radiology, St. George's Hospital, London, UK

A. England
Department of Radiography, University of Salford, Manchester, UK

K. Flood
Department of Vascular Radiology,
Leeds General Infirmary, Leeds, UK

M.-F. Giroux
Department of Radiology, CHUM-Centre Hospitalier
de l'Université de Montréal, Montreal, QC, Canada

R.G. McWilliams
Department of Radiology, Royal Liverpool
University Hospital, Liverpool, UK

J.V. Patel
Department of Radiology, The Leeds Teaching
Hospitals NHS Trust, Leeds, West Yorkshire, UK

R. Patel
Department of Radiology,
The Leeds Teaching Hospitals NHS Trust,
Leeds, West Yorkshire, UK
e-mail: rafpatel@gmail.com

U. Patel
Department of Diagnostic Radiology,
St. George's Hospital and Medical School,
Blackshaw Road, SW17 0QT London, UK
e-mail: uday.patel@stgeorges.nhs.uk

L. Ratnam
Department of Radiology, St. George's Hospital,
Blackshaw Road, SW17 0QT London, UK
e-mail: lakshmi.ratnam@nhs.net

R.P. Yadavali
Department of Radiology, Aberdeen Royal
Infirmary, Aberdeen, UK

J. Rose
Department of Interventional Radiology,
Freeman Hospital, Newcastle Upon Tyne Hospitals
NHS Trust, Newcastle upon Tyne, UK

Chapter 27. Protrusion of Vena Cava Filter into the Aorta

Case History

An 18-year-old female was referred to our institution for retrieval of an inferior vena cava (IVC) filter. She had a Celect (Cook) filter placed 8 months previously in another hospital. A pre-procedure portal venous CT was obtained (Fig. 27.1), and the filter was seen to have perforated through the cava and possibly through the aorta.

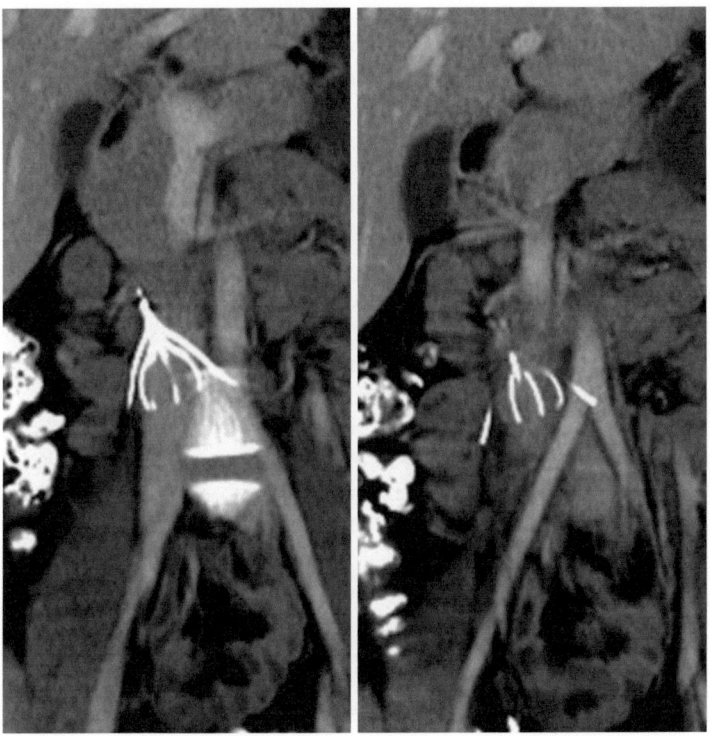

FIGURE 27.1 Portal venous phase CT demonstrating a tilted IVC filter, abutting the lateral wall of the vein. Some struts are protruding outside the confines of the vena cava. More specifically, one of the left legs had also transgressed the right lateral wall of the infrarenal aorta, at the aortic bifurcation. There was no retroperitoneal bleeding or aortic pseudoaneurysm

Procedure

As this patient was very young, it was decided to attempt removal of the filter. Before the procedure, it was ensured that arterial vascular occlusion balloons and proper stent grafts were available in the event of aortic hemorrhage, and the vascular surgery team were consulted and forewarned.

The procedure was initiated with right internal jugular vein access, and classic attempts at filter removal with the use of different snares and recovery cone were unsuccessful. A second puncture of the right internal jugular vein was undertaken, and snaring of the entire filter was attempted, using a reverse curve catheter. The curve was formed below the stent struts in the hope that the filter could be mobilized and to free the hook from the caval wall.

This technique also failed. Therefore, a right femoral vein access was used as well. There were many attempts at liberating the hook from the caval wall, by introducing an 8 mm × 40 mm angioplasty balloon between the two structures, from cephalad and caudal approaches. There was also a simultaneous attempt as a second interventional radiologist tried seizing the removal hook from the jugular access (Fig. 27.2).

After 5 unsuccessful hours, filter removal attempt was abandoned. The patient recovered uneventfully and was discharged within 24 h. Because of the patient's age, it was decided by the referring team not to give long-term anticoagulation to this patient.

Discussion

IVC filters have evolved in the last decade and most devices are now retrievable. However, the filters are still prone to tilting and the struts can penetrate through the caval wall. Tilting also favors incorporation of the cephalad tip into the caval wall. This tip being the key to the removal of the most commonly used retrievable filters; its incorporation may prevent removal of the filter. Many techniques have been described, including those illustrated and used here: double

Chapter 27. Protrusion of Vena Cava Filter into the Aorta 209

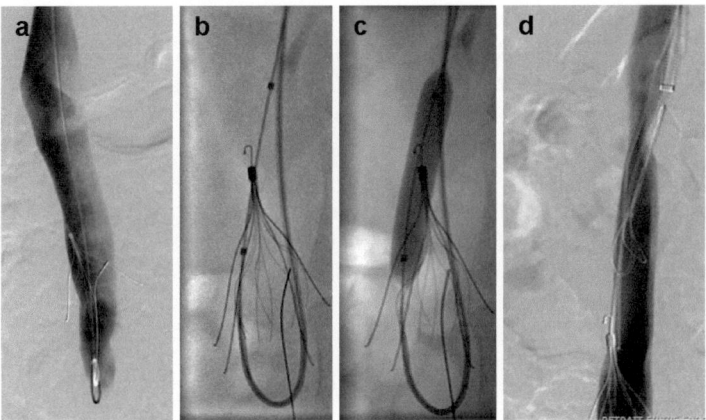

FIGURE 27.2 (**a–d**) Montage of the various maneuvers used to free an incorporated tip and legs of an IVC filter from the walls of the inferior vena cava. Neither the snare loop (**b**) nor balloon (**c**) succeeded in mobilizing the filter

venous access, loop technique, snares, balloons, photothermal ablation, forceps, etc.

Obviously, the most important way to prevent retrieval problems is to follow proper guidelines at insertion. Firstly, the indication for the filter should be adequate. The filter should be well positioned and not tilted as this will facilitate successful retrieval. Follow-up of the patients with proposed temporary filters is also very important, as this will permit optimization of the timing for retrieval. The filter should be retrieved as soon as it is no longer necessary, as the longer its parts lay against the caval wall, the greater the risks of incorporation.

Tips

- If feasible, filter deployment should favor the hook to be away from caval wall.
- Deployment of the filter legs should not be into major/visible veins (e.g., renal or lumbar) as this predisposes to filter tilting.

- All patients with optional filters implanted should be followed up. Reasons for non-retrieval (if so desired for medical reasons) should be documented in the patients' charts. All other patients should be considered for retrieval, investigated as such, and have a reasonable attempt at filter retrieval.
- Never forget that these filters are optional and can be left permanently if the risks of retrieval are deemed higher than benefits.

Commentary

Retrievable (or optional) IVC filters are designed for short-term use but can be left permanently. The manufacturers recommend retrieval within 6 weeks of insertion, although there are reports of successful retrieval as long as 180 days or more after insertion. Naturally, the longer they are left in place, the more difficult they are to remove, as the legs or the tip becomes incorporated into the wall. It is also not uncommon for the struts to penetrate through the caval wall, although this in itself is seldom of clinical importance.

Failure is more common in those with longer dwell times, increasing age of patient, incorporation of the struts into the wall, and filter tilt, although the latter was not considered an impediment in one large study.

The simplest method is to snare the hook at the cephalad tip and lift the filter free from the wall. If this fails, usually because the hook cannot be engaged because the filter is tilted, then a snare loop can be formed underneath the filter, between the struts and legs, using either a wire and snare, or a catheter and snare. Once the loop is formed and as it is withdrawn, the filter will be lifted free off the wall. Care is necessary as the struts may fracture. Balloon dilatation may help. As the balloon is dilated, the walls of the IVC are pulled away and the tip or legs will be freed off the wall.

But sometimes none of these tricks work, in which case the filter can be left in situ. The long-term outcome of IVC filters is still unknown, and so follow-up may be prudent.

Further Reading

Caplin DM, Nikolic B, Kalva SP, Ganguli S, et al. Quality improvement guidelines for the performance of inferior vena cava filter placement for the prevention of pulmonary embolism. J Vasc Interv Radiol. 2011;22(11):1499–506.

Marquess JS, Burke CT, Beecham AH, Dixon RG, et al. Factors associated with failed retrieval of the Günther Tulip inferior vena cava filter. J Vasc Interv Radiol. 2008;19:1321–7.

Chapter 28
The Multiple Options for Retrieval of a Tilted IVC Filter

Robert P. Allison, Anna Maria Belli, Joo-Young Chun, Raymond Chung, Raj Das, Andrew England, Karen Flood, Marie-France Giroux, Richard G. McWilliams, Robert Morgan, Nik Papadakos, Jai V. Patel, Raf Patel, Uday Patel, Lakshmi Ratnam, Reddi Prasad Yadavali, and John Rose

Abstract This case describes a range of maneuvers utilized in an attempt to straighten an IVC filter tilted into a lumbar vein. The technical description is accompanied by images of the various techniques.

Keywords IVC filter retrieval • Complications • Tilting • Snare • Angioplasty balloon

R.P. Allison
Department of Interventional Radiology,
University Hospitals Southampton,
Southampton, Hampshire, UK

A.M. Belli
Department of Radiology, St. George's Hospital and Medical School, Blackshaw Road,
London SW17 0RE, UK
e-mail: anna.belli@stgeorges.nhs.uk

J.-Y. Chun • R. Chung • R. Das • R. Morgan • N. Papadakos
Department of Radiology, St. George's Hospital,
London, UK

A. England
Department of Radiography, University of Salford,
Manchester, UK

K. Flood
Department of Vascular Radiology,
Leeds General Infirmary, Leeds, UK

M.-F. Giroux
Department of Radiology, CHUM-Centre Hospitalier
de l'Université de Montréal, Montreal, QC, Canada

R.G. McWilliams
Department of Radiology, Royal Liverpool
University Hospital, Liverpool, UK

J.V. Patel
Department of Radiology, The Leeds Teaching
Hospitals NHS Trust, Leeds, West Yorkshire, UK

R. Patel
Department of Radiology,
The Leeds Teaching Hospitals NHS Trust,
Leeds, West Yorkshire, UK
e-mail: rafpatel@gmail.com

U. Patel
Department of Diagnostic Radiology,
St. George's Hospital and Medical School,
Blackshaw Road, SW17 0QT London, UK
e-mail: uday.patel@stgeorges.nhs.uk

L. Ratnam
Department of Radiology, St. George's Hospital,
Blackshaw Road, SW17 0QT London, UK
e-mail: lakshmi.ratnam@nhs.net

R.P. Yadavali
Department of Radiology, Aberdeen Royal
Infirmary, Aberdeen, UK

J. Rose
Department of Interventional Radiology,
Freeman Hospital, Newcastle Upon Tyne
Hospitals NHS Trust, Newcastle upon Tyne, UK

Case History

A 49-year-old male with chronic renal insufficiency and renal transplant presented with cardiac arrhythmias and was found to have deep venous thrombosis and pulmonary emboli. Less than a month later, he presented again with abdominal pain, found to be due to gangrenous calculous cholecystitis requiring surgery. The surgeon and nephrologist considered the patient as having a temporary contraindication to anticoagulation and requested insertion of an optional inferior vena cava (IVC) filter. A Recovery (Bard) filter was uneventfully positioned (Fig. 28.1) in an infrarenal location by a right common femoral approach. Three weeks after successful surgery, filter removal was requested.

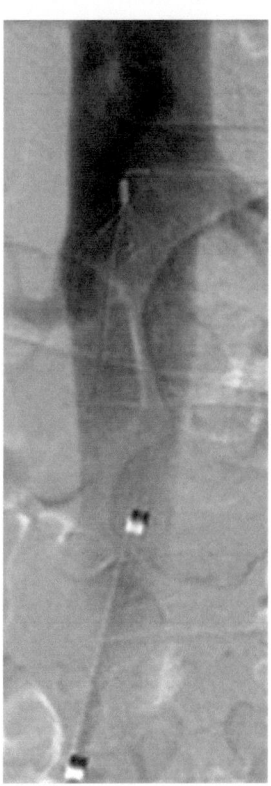

FIGURE 28.1 A well-positioned and well-orientated IVC filter

Procedure

At initial cavogram, the filter was in a good position for retrieval (Fig. 28.2). Unfortunately during exchange of the flush catheter for the retrieval sheath, the apex of the filter tilted laterally into a lumbar vein, with one of the arms deformed. Passage of a wire on the right lateral side of the vena cava and angioplasty, with traction of the balloon, to displace the apex of the filter out of the lumbar vein was unsuccessful (Fig. 28.2); as were attempts to capture the apex with a small snare and traction to pull the apex out of the lumbar vein (Fig. 28.2) resulting in an asymptomatic venous dissection.

Further attempts at retrieval were postponed for 5 days. At second attempt, a loop-snare technique by the femoral approach was first used (Fig. 28.3) to try to straighten the filter. This resulted in the filter not reerecting but deforming drastically as it struck a ballet pose (the splits) – Fig. 28.3b. Then, there was an attempt at using a trilobed snare from a right internal jugular vein access, as upward pressure was applied on the apex from below with an angioplasty balloon (Fig. 28.3).

Finally, a similar technique to the last one but using a recovery cone instead of the snare proved to be the right combination for this patient. It permitted the capture of the

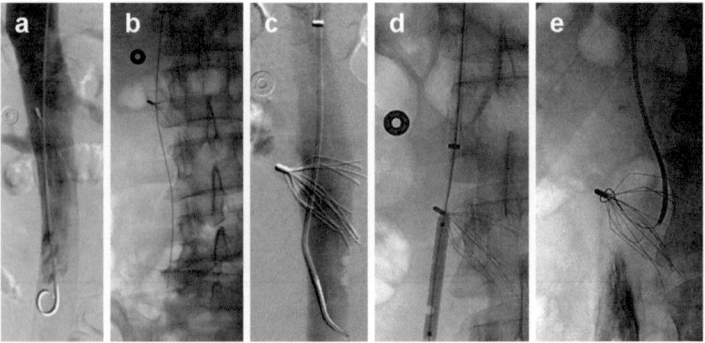

FIGURE 28.2 (**a**–**e**) The initial venogram shows a well-orientated IVC filter. On catheter removal the filter has tilted, and its tip is now in a branch vein (**c**). (**d**, **e**) show that neither a balloon nor a snare was able to reorientate the filter for retrieval. Venous dissection is seen in (**e**)

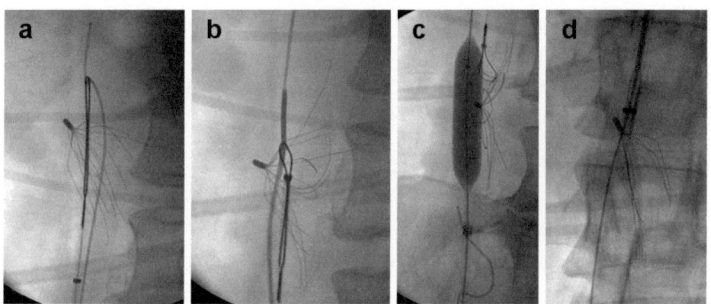

FIGURE 28.3 Combined femoral and jugular approaches. In (**a**, **b**) a loop-snare technique merely worsens the orientation of the legs. In (**c**) a balloon has been inserted from the femoral route and inflated below the filter and pushed superiorly while the filter is snared using a trilobed snare inserted by the jugular route. This failed, but once the snare was replaced with a recovery cone, (**d**) the filter was straightened into the IVC. It was then removed using standard snaring technique of the tip

junction between the apex and the struts. Pulling with the cone straightened the filter back into the caval lumen, making it possible to release the apex-struts junction from the cone and recapturing the apex itself, finalizing the procedure in its usual manner. The final cavogram revealed no significant abnormality, the filter was intact at visual inspection, and the patient had a good clinical course.

Discussion

Optional IVC filters are now very commonly used and removed. The main problem encountered at retrieval is tilting, with or without caval wall tip incorporation. In this case, as the tilt resulted from a technical error, we were assured that the apex of the filter was not embedded in the venous wall. This encouraged us to be more aggressive in our retrieval attempts since the risks of ripping the caval wall was lessened, though not absent. There are different techniques that have and could have been used.

First, trial of simple, conventional procedures should always be considered, as the risks of complications are low.

These options include the use of standard snares, multiple lobe snares, and recovery cones.

Then, if geometry prevents success, variants of such conventional techniques are used. These include:

1. Mobilization of the filter apex by the "twist technique," in which the superior part of the filter is engaged with a reversed curve catheter and its apex is re-centered as the catheter is slightly, gently rotated and pulled.
2. Modified snare technique, in which the snare is introduced into a curved catheter to help direct it towards the filter apex.
3. Loop-snare technique, which has been extensively described. This procedure involves looping a wire around the superior part of the filter, from a jugular access, snaring the wire from the jugular access and advancing the jugular sheath over this homemade snare, to recapture the filter.
4. Balloon-assisted technique, which uses an inflated angioplasty balloon introduced between the filter apex and the caval wall to deflect the apex. This can be used from a jugular and/or femoral access, before or during the attempt at capturing the apex.
5. Use of different types of forceps to mobilize the apex of the filter.

Tips

- Knowing the apex of the filter is not embedded in a vessel wall can justify a more aggressive retrieval attempt.
- Always make sure all the arms, legs, apex, and leg hooks of the filter are complete once the filter is removed, as difficult retrievals often lead to pieces breaking off the filter.
- Many unsuccessful retrieval attempts in non-incorporated filters are due to geometrical problems and can be solved by using variants of conventional techniques.
- In these modified techniques, make sure to do no harm by manipulating carefully, as not to break pieces off the filter, snares, wires, and catheters.
- Also, you have to prevent the different tools from being permanently caught in a filter that you might not be able to remove.

Commentary

There are many lessons in this case. Foremost being the ease with which a filter may be dislodged and the difficulty posed if the tip has protruded into a branch vein. The authors also describe a stepwise, intelligent approach to the problem of the tilted filter. The simplest and first approach should be the use of the various snares and recovery cones to correct the tilt. If that fails, then various shaped catheters or balloons or loop snares are used. If these fail, then the filter may have to be left as a permanent filter.

In this case tilting occurred during retrieval, and protrusion into a branch vein is a recognized cause. In this case the filter protruded into a lumbar vein, but this can happen into the renal, hepatic, or gonadal veins. Critical tilting is defined as the filter axis being >15° compared to the axis of the vena cava. It most commonly occurs during filter insertion, in between 1 and 5 % of cases, and as well as making retrieval difficult, it is believed to reduce filtering efficiency and also to increase the risk of caval wall perforation. Tilting is a perennial problem affecting all filter designs. Design modifications have failed to eliminate the risk, but it may be more common after left femoral vein access, and there are described technical maneuvers that may reduce the risk (see under further reading).

Further Reading

Knott EM, Beacham B, Fry WR. New technique to prevent tilt during inferior vena cava filter placement. J Vasc Surg. 2012;55(3):869–71.

Lynch FC. Balloon-assisted removal of tilted inferior vena cava filters with embedded tips. J Vasc Interv Radiol. 2009;20:1210–24.

Van Ha TG, Vinokur O, Lorenz J, Regalado S, et al. Techniques used for difficult retrievals of the Günther Tulip inferior vena cava filter: experience in 32 patients. J Vasc Interv Radiol. 2009;20:92–9.

Chapter 29
Retrieval of a Well-Orientated IVC Filter with Embedded Struts

Robert P. Allison, Anna Maria Belli, Joo-Young Chun, Raymond Chung, Raj Das, Andrew England, Karen Flood, Marie-France Giroux, Richard G. McWilliams, Robert Morgan, Nik Papadakos, Jai V. Patel, Raf Patel, Uday Patel, Lakshmi Ratnam, Reddi Prasad Yadavali, and John Rose

Abstract This case describes the retrieval of an IVC filter in which the struts had become embedded in the caval wall. Balloon angioplasty and combined jugular and femoral access are utilized to free the filter prior to retrieval.

Keywords IVC filter retrieval • Complications • Embedded • Incorporated

---

R.P. Allison
Department of Interventional Radiology,
University Hospitals Southampton,
Southampton, Hampshire, UK

A.M. Belli
Department of Radiology, St. George's Hospital and Medical School, Blackshaw Road,
London SW17 0RE, UK
e-mail: anna.belli@stgeorges.nhs.uk

J.-Y. Chun • R. Chung • R. Das • R. Morgan • N. Papadakos
Department of Radiology, St. George's Hospital, London, UK

A. England
Department of Radiography, University of Salford, Manchester, UK

K. Flood
Department of Vascular Radiology,
Leeds General Infirmary, Leeds, UK

M.-F. Giroux
Department of Radiology, CHUM-Centre Hospitalier
de l'Université de Montréal, Montreal, QC, Canada

R.G. McWilliams
Department of Radiology, Royal Liverpool
University Hospital, Liverpool, UK

J.V. Patel
Department of Radiology, The Leeds Teaching
Hospitals NHS Trust, Leeds, West Yorkshire, UK

R. Patel
Department of Radiology,
The Leeds Teaching Hospitals NHS Trust,
Leeds, West Yorkshire, UK
e-mail: rafpatel@gmail.com

U. Patel
Department of Diagnostic Radiology,
St. George's Hospital and Medical School,
Blackshaw Road, SW17 0QT London, UK
e-mail: uday.patel@stgeorges.nhs.uk

L. Ratnam
Department of Radiology, St. George's Hospital,
Blackshaw Road, SW17 0QT London, UK
e-mail: lakshmi.ratnam@nhs.net

R.P. Yadavali
Department of Radiology, Aberdeen Royal
Infirmary, Aberdeen, UK

J. Rose
Department of Interventional Radiology,
Freeman Hospital, Newcastle Upon Tyne
Hospitals NHS Trust, Newcastle upon Tyne, UK

Case History

A 72-year-old female was admitted with deep venous thrombosis of the lower extremity, complicated by pulmonary embolism. Despite therapeutic anticoagulation with warfarin, she developed bilateral adrenal hematoma, precluding the continuation of anticoagulation. Therefore, a Celect (Cook) inferior vena cava (IVC) filter was inserted. Four months later, anticoagulation could be resumed, and interventional radiology was consulted for removal of the filter.

Procedure

Initial cavogram shows the filter to be upright, without any tilting or clot entrapment. However, extensive intimal hyperplasia had occurred, engulfing at least two of the filter legs and incorporating them into the vessel wall (Fig. 29.1a), almost along their entire length. Retrieval was nevertheless attempted. First, balloon angioplasty was used to separate vessel wall from the legs as much as possible (Fig. 29.1b). Then, a trilobed snare was used to grasp the top hook (Fig. 29.1c). With traction on the snare, the retrieval sheath was finally advanced slowly over the filter, creating a blunt dissection around the collapsing filter (Fig. 29.1d). Notice that a venous femoral access sheath was also in place to permit rapid balloon introduction should IVC rupture occur, in the hope of permitting tamponade of the bleed.

Final cavogram (Fig. 29.1e) shows secondary dissection of the IVC once the filter was removed. There was also a small amount of clot secondary to the procedure. The patient remained on therapeutic anticoagulation and without any sequelae.

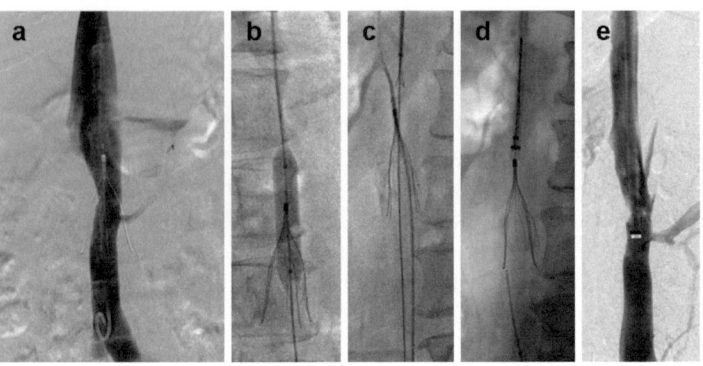

FIGURE 29.1 (**a**) Shows a well-orientated filter, but the struts (or legs) are incorporated into the walls of the IVC. Technical difficulty was anticipated, and a combined femoral and jugular approach was selected. (**b**) Balloon angioplasty was undertaken to free the legs from the wall. (**c, d**) Then the filter tip was captured via the jugular route and the filter removed (see text). (**e**) Some minor clot but no major extravasation. Note that the femoral access would have allowed the rapid introduction of a tamponade balloon in the case of major venous leak or rupture

Discussion

With optional filters, retrieval, tilting, and/or incorporation of filter parts are the most prevalent problems encountered. Embedding of the tip is most problematic as it prevents capture of the hook at the tip for removal. But, incorporation of the arms and legs can also lead to difficult retrieval, as these parts may not collapse properly into the retrieval sheath. Increased force has to be applied on the filter in this setting, increasing the risks of filter fracture and venous injuries such as caval rupture, dissection, invagination, and clot formation. Commonly abdominal pain is experienced during removal.

One of the main factors for filter incorporation is indwelling time. Therefore, time between installation and retrieval should be minimized if clinically feasible. Also, and most noteworthy, patients with optional filters should be kept track of by the interventional radiology team.

Once the filter is partly incorporated in the caval wall, options for retrieval are reduced. Besides the use of force, some teams have started using metallic forceps, permitting dissection around the incorporated part of the filter, mostly described for incorporation of the tip. Also, more recently, some teams have used a laser-assisted sheath technique.

After such forceful and/or complex manipulations, visual filter inspection for missing pieces should be part of the routine. In addition, final IVC imaging is essential as injuries to the vessel should be documented and addressed immediately, even though most of the time, the treatment will be conservative. Of course, IVC rupture, which is exceedingly rare, would require immediate treatment, most probably with balloon tamponade and possible stent grafting. However, much more commonly, there will be less important wall injury such as dissection or clot formation. These two can usually be managed solely with systemic anticoagulation.

Tips

- Final cavogram post-filter retrieval or retrieval attempt is mandatory.
- Complications of retrieval attempts such as IVC dissection/stenosis and clot formation are usually managed conservatively, without long-term consequences.
- Filter material might change your approach to filter retrieval in case of incorporated parts, as elastic metals can be deformed and therefore manipulated more extensively with less caval injury.

Commentary

Neovascularization can very rapidly engulf the struts of an IVC filter. In such cases, difficult filter retrieval can be anticipated. A combined femoral and jugular approach should be considered. This increases the range of maneuvers available for retrieval but will also allow for the rapid introduction of a tamponade balloon in the case of catastrophic venous damage.

Initial balloon dilatation of the IVC helps free and mobilize the legs, but this should be undertaken with care as the balloon can become entrapped in the filter. In fact any device can become entrapped by the filters' legs and arms and should be used with care.

Further Reading

Kuo WT, Tong RT, Hwang GL, Louie JD, et al. High-risk retrieval of adherent and chronically implanted IVC filters: techniques for removal and management of thrombotic complications. J Vasc Interv Radiol. 2009;20:1548–56.

Lyon SM, Riojas GE, Uberoi R, Patel J, et al. Short- and long-term retrievability of the Celect vena cava filter: results of a multi-institutional registry. J Vasc Interv Radiol. 2009;20:1441–8.

Chapter 30
Retrieving a Tilted IVC Filter with Struts Penetrating the IVC

Robert P. Allison, Anna Maria Belli, Joo-Young Chun, Raymond Chung, Raj Das, Andrew England, Karen Flood, Marie-France Giroux, Richard G. McWilliams, Robert Morgan, Nik Papadakos, Jai V. Patel, Raf Patel, Uday Patel, Lakshmi Ratnam, Reddi Prasad Yadavali, and John Rose

Abstract This case illustrates retrieval of a suprarenal IVC filter which had tilted significantly with embedding of the filter struts into the caval wall.

Keywords IVC filter retrieval • Complications • Tilting • Embedded • Snare

---

R.P. Allison
Department of Interventional Radiology, University Hospitals Southampton, Southampton, Hampshire, UK

A.M. Belli
Department of Radiology, St. George's Hospital
and Medical School, Blackshaw Road,
London SW17 0RE, UK
e-mail: anna.belli@stgeorges.nhs.uk

J.-Y. Chun • R. Chung • R. Das • R. Morgan • N. Papadakos
Department of Radiology, St. George's Hospital, London, UK

A. England
Department of Radiography, University of Salford, Manchester, UK

K. Flood
Department of Vascular Radiology,
Leeds General Infirmary, Leeds, UK

M.-F. Giroux
Department of Radiology, CHUM-Centre Hospitalier
de l'Université de Montréal, Montreal, QC, Canada

R.G. McWilliams
Department of Radiology, Royal Liverpool
University Hospital, Liverpool, UK

J.V. Patel
Department of Radiology, The Leeds Teaching
Hospitals NHS Trust, Leeds, West Yorkshire, UK

R. Patel
Department of Radiology,
The Leeds Teaching Hospitals NHS Trust,
Leeds, West Yorkshire, UK
e-mail: rafpatel@gmail.com

U. Patel
Department of Diagnostic Radiology,
St. George's Hospital and Medical School,
Blackshaw Road, SW17 0QT London, UK
e-mail: uday.patel@stgeorges.nhs.uk

L. Ratnam
Department of Radiology, St. George's Hospital,
Blackshaw Road, SW17 0QT London, UK
e-mail: lakshmi.ratnam@nhs.net

R.P. Yadavali
Department of Radiology, Aberdeen Royal
Infirmary, Aberdeen, UK

J. Rose
Department of Interventional Radiology,
Freeman Hospital, Newcastle Upon Tyne
Hospitals NHS Trust, Newcastle upon Tyne, UK

Case History

A 54-year-old male with a past history of pulmonary emboli was admitted with right lower limb ischemia. A CT angiogram was obtained demonstrating underlying atheromatous disease, with in situ thrombosis of the right popliteal artery and emboli in the lower leg arteries. Extensive venous thrombosis of the same limb was also discovered, with extension into the femoral and iliac veins (Fig. 30.1a) and possibly into the inferior vena cava. The surgical team requested the insertion of an inferior vena cava (IVC) filter to stop the systemic anticoagulation. Therefore, a Recovery (Bard) filter was placed.

Procedure

Because of the right iliac deep vein thrombus (DVT), a left femoral vein approach was used and venography confirmed IVC clot (Fig. 30.1b, c). It was decided to insert the filter from a right internal jugular vein approach to prevent clot manipulation and possible embolization. Unfortunately, the clot extended to the renal veins, and there was very little distance between the renal veins and the atrio-caval junction. Therefore, the filter was positioned above the renal veins, but the legs and arms were all close to or in front of

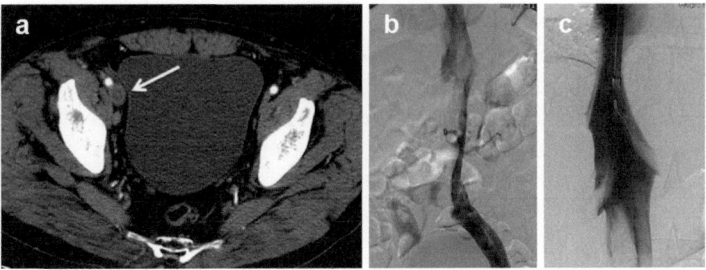

FIGURE 30.1 (a) Thrombosis in the right external iliac vein (*arrow*); (b, c) extension up to the infrarenal IVC

the renal veins as the filter apex would have been in the atrium if the filter had been positioned more cephalad. It was recommended that the filter be retrieved as soon as possible to prevent renal vein thrombosis and filter migration into the heart.

Unfortunately, filter extraction was requested over 9 months later, with the patient already under anticoagulation (Fig. 30.2). The initial cavogram shows a severely tilted filter, with wall penetration of many filter legs and arms but the IVC clot had cleared. Retrieval was first attempted by positioning a guidewire between the filter apex and the cava wall ("on the short side," to use the common terminology of many interventional radiologists) and passing the retrieval cone on the wire to grab the top of the filter. This proved unsuccessful and the "balloon technique" was attempted, also with failure. The "side-branch technique," which is catheterizing a side branch close to the filter apex and using a snare within the branch to grab the filter apex, was also tried without success. Finally, the "catheter-snare technique" proved useful as it permitted straightening of the filter and proper retrieval.

Discussion

In this specific case, large clot burden prevented infrarenal positioning of the filter. However, once a filter is placed, clot will not necessarily impede subsequent filter ensnarement and retrieval as by the time of retrieval it can be expected to have dissolved.

Sometimes, the tilted apex of the filter is adjacent to a venous tributary of the IVC. In addition to the conventional techniques for mobilizing the filter tip (twist, modified snare, loop snare, balloon-assisted techniques, and forceps use), this situation permits the use of another maneuver, the "branch technique," whereby the branch vein in which the tip lies is cannulated with the snare open and the tip ensnared. This will straighten the filter. Retrieval can then proceed as per normal.

Chapter 30. Tilted IVC Filter with Embedded Struts

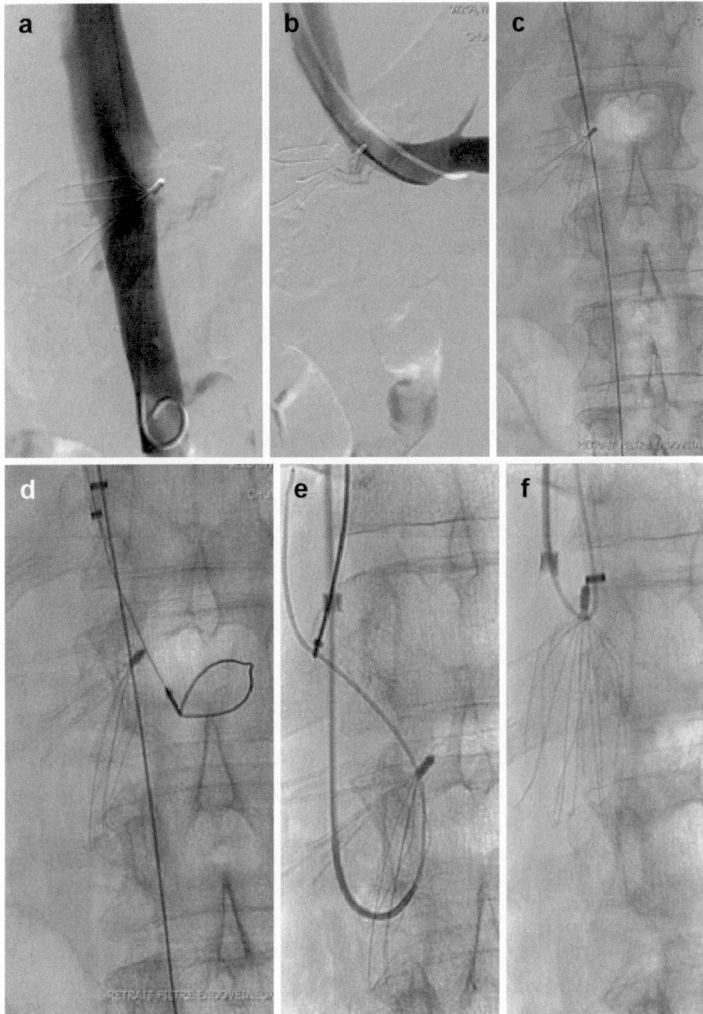

FIGURE 30.2 (**a, b**) Show the IVC filter has tilted with the tip in the left renal vein. A guidewire/retrieval cone ensemble failed to grasp the filter apex (**c**). The left renal vein was catheterized (side-branch technique) with a snare loop (**d**), but this failed to reorientate the filter. (**e, f**) show the "catheter-snare" technique which successfully straightened the filter tip and allowed filter retrieval

Tips

- Reviewing images from previous examinations, especially abdominal/pelvic CT and MR provide important information to plan the filter placement (site of clots/thromboses, accessory renal veins, etc.).
- Filter penetration is rarely an issue but some associated complications have been described such as retroperitoneal hemorrhage and other organ penetration (aorta, duodenum, ureters, and pancreas).
- Rarely, filter penetration, without any complication, can be associated with abdominal pain.
- Clot entrapment in the filter rarely prevents eventual retrieval of the filter, as most patients kept on anticoagulation will lyse the clot.
- During filter placement, if feasible, installation of the legs at the level of vena cava tributaries should be avoided as it may promote filter tilting.

Commentary

Although suprarenal positioning of IVC filters is an accepted technique, it should be used only when indicated, e.g., extensive clot in the infrarenal IVC, complex venous anomalies such as a dual IVC or when the renal vein is thrombosed, e.g., with renal cell carcinoma. In all such cases, careful placement is crucial. The ideal location is between the renal veins and the hepatic vein confluence, but as this case illustrates, this can be challenging and either tilting or protrusion into a branch vein is a constant concern.

Accurate placement is facilitated by good planning venography, which should ideally demonstrate both the left and right renal veins as well as the hepatic vein confluence. There is also a greater risk of migration, and this can be into the right atrium or even the pulmonary artery. The latter two require particularly well-planned retrieval, and a method of approach is listed under further reading.

Further Reading

Iliescu B, Haskal ZJ. Advanced techniques for removal of retrievable vena cava filters. Cardiovasc Intervent Radiol. 2012;35(4):741–50.

Kaufman JA, Kinney TB, Streiff MB, Sing RF, et al. Guidelines for the use of retrievable and convertible vena cava filters: report from the Society of Interventional Radiology multidisciplinary consensus conference. J Vasc Interv Radiol. 2006;17:449–59.

Oliva VL, Perreault P, Giroux M-F, Bouchard L, et al. Recovery G2 inferior vena cava filter: technical success and safety of retrieval. J Vasc Interv Radiol. 2008;19:884–9.

Owens CA, Bui JT, Knuttinen MG, Gaba RC, Carrillo TC, Gast T. Endovascular retrieval of intracardiac inferior vena cava filters: a review of published techniques. J Vasc Interv Radiol. 2009;20(11):1418–28.

Chapter 31
Fistula Rupture Post-fistuloplasty

Robert P. Allison, Anna Maria Belli, Joo-Young Chun, Raymond Chung, Raj Das, Andrew England, Karen Flood, Marie-France Giroux, Richard G. kMcWilliams, Robert Morgan, Nik Papadakos, Jai V. Patel, Raf Patel, Uday Patel, Lakshmi Ratnam, Reddi Prasad Yadavali, and John Rose

Abstract This case outlines management of rupture of an arteriovenous fistula following balloon dilatation of a stenosis with a cutting balloon. Clinical and technical tips are provided for dealing with such a situation acutely.

Keywords Fistuloplasty • Complications • Rupture • Stent

R.P. Allison
Department of Interventional Radiology,
University Hospitals Southampton,
Southampton, Hampshire, UK

A.M. Belli
Department of Radiology, St. George's Hospital
and Medical School, Blackshaw Road,
London, SW17 0RE, UK
e-mail: anna.belli@stgeorges.nhs.uk

J.-Y. Chun • R. Chung
R. Das • R. Morgan • N. Papadakos
Department of Radiology, St. George's
Hospital, London, UK

A. England
Department of Radiography, University of Salford, Manchester, UK

K. Flood
Department of Vascular Radiology,
Leeds General Infirmary, Leeds, UK

M.-F. Giroux
Department of Radiology, CHUM-Centre
Hospitalier de l'Université de Montréal,
Montreal, QC, Canada

R.G. McWilliams
Department of Radiology, Royal Liverpool
University Hospital, Liverpool, UK

J.V. Patel
Department of Radiology, The Leeds Teaching
Hospitals NHS Trust, Leeds, West Yorkshire, UK

R. Patel
Department of Radiology,
The Leeds Teaching Hospitals NHS Trust,
Leeds, West Yorkshire, UK
e-mail: rafpatel@gmail.com

U. Patel
Department of Diagnostic Radiology,
St. George's Hospital and Medical School,
Blackshaw Road, SW17 0QT London, UK
e-mail: uday.patel@stgeorges.nhs.uk

L. Ratnam
Department of Radiology, St. George's Hospital,
Blackshaw Road, SW17 0QT London, UK
e-mail: lakshmi.ratnam@nhs.net

R.P. Yadavali
Department of Radiology, Aberdeen Royal
Infirmary, Aberdeen, UK

J. Rose
Department of Interventional Radiology,
Freeman Hospital, Newcastle Upon Tyne
Hospitals NHS Trust, Newcastle upon Tyne, UK

Case History

A 79-year-old man with end-stage renal failure attended for a fistulogram of his poorly functioning left brachio-basilic arteriovenous fistula. Poor flows during dialysis had prompted a duplex ultrasound scan, which demonstrated >75 % stenosis in the basilic vein.

Procedure

Diagnostic fistulography confirmed a long stenosis in the draining vein (Fig. 31.1a). The arterial anastomosis and central veins were patent. The stenosis was suitable for angioplasty.

The stenosis was crossed with a guidewire, and a 6 mm cutting balloon was used for primary angioplasty. The waist of the balloon was successfully abolished. However, on check venography, there was clear evidence of a venous leak in keeping with vessel rupture and acute extravasation (Fig. 31.1b). Initially, a standard 8 mm angioplasty balloon was inserted across the rupture site and left inflated for 5–10 min as a means of tamponade. This failed to stop the extravasation, and therefore, an 8 mm stent graft was deployed across the rupture. Hemostasis was achieved with good flow within the fistula and no evidence of persisting stenosis post procedure (Fig. 31.1c).

Discussion

Dialysis fistulas are prone to stenosis, and treatment is recommended when they reduce dialysis efficiency. Angioplasty will successfully treat most stenosis, but these can be resistant to standard balloon angioplasty. High-pressure balloons or cutting balloons become necessary.

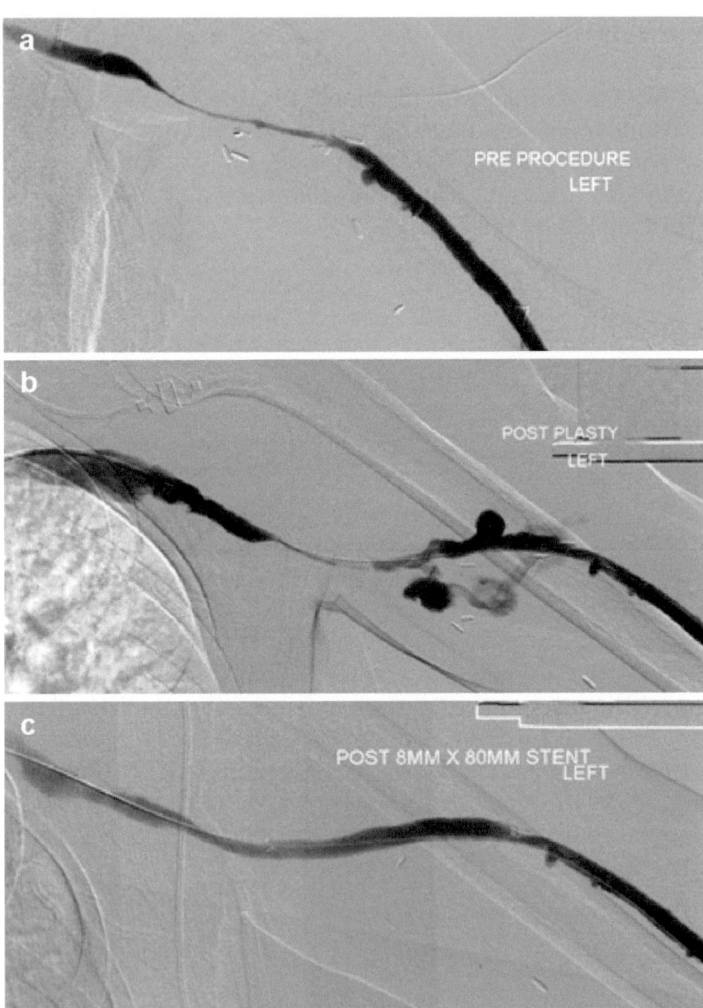

FIGURE 31.1 (**a**) Diagnostic fistulogram demonstrating long, tight stenosis of the axillary vein; (**b**) venogram postprimary cutting balloon angioplasty demonstrating venous rupture; (**c**) hemostasis post stent deployment

Cutting balloons are noncompliant balloons with three to four microsurgical blades (atherotomes) mounted longitudinally that project 0.1 mm on inflation, incising the fibroelastic neointimal hyperplasia in a controlled manner. Slow smooth inflation/deflation of these balloons is advised to allow the atherotomes to deploy without risking the integrity of the balloon itself. Further dilatation can then be achieved at lower pressures with a standard angioplasty balloon if required. The results from cutting balloon angioplasty are as good as and possibly better than that achieved with standard balloon dilatation. Wu et al. reported a slightly higher primary patency at 6-month follow-up in the cohort undergoing cutting balloon angioplasty, with primary patency rates of 71.4 % at 6 months compared to 42.9 %, in the high-pressure balloon angioplasty group.

Cutting balloons are prone to similar complications as conventional balloon angioplasty such as vessel rupture, dissection, and pseudoaneurysm formation with reported complication rates from 0 to 5.2 %. In addition, blade dislodgement is a possibility and best avoided by slow, controlled inflation/deflation. Increased chance of vessel rupture has been described if used immediately after standard balloon angioplasty, and some recommend the use of cutting balloons as primary treatment or prior to larger-diameter standard balloon angioplasty.

Depending on the degree of extravasation, this can be treated either by manual compression, endovascular balloon compression, or stenting. However, the long-term patency of the vascular access is thought suboptimal.

Tips

- For resistant stenoses, primary treatment with cutting balloon angioplasty is suggested.
- In the case of failed initial standard balloon angioplasty, further use of cutting balloon may increase the risk of vessel rupture.
- Stenting in venous rupture, although at times unavoidable, is better left as a last resort.

Commentary

Thrombosis and vessel rupture are the most serious complications encountered during dialysis fistula intervention. Rupture may be heralded by an audible pop or increased pain and swelling of the arm. In which case, the degree of extravasation should be assessed. Minor, contained leak may not require any further management. A greater leak should be first treated with balloon tamponade. A long balloon left inflated across the rupture for a period of 10 min may seal the leak. Some have advocated that 3×10-min inflations should be tried before this is deemed a failure, but this was in the past and before the ready availability of covered stents. While the balloon is left inflated, the fistula should be kept regularly flushed with saline to avoid proximal thrombosis. Anecdotal evidence suggests that ruptures after cutting balloon angioplasty are long linear tears and that balloon tamponade is less likely to succeed.

If simple tamponade fails, the only other option is a covered stent or a stent graft, although bare stents have been used with variable success for this purpose.

Further Reading

Aruny JE, Lewis CA, Cardella JF, et al. Quality improvement guidelines for percutaneous management of the thrombosed or dysfunctional dialysis access. Standards of Practice Committee of the Society of Cardiovascular and Interventional Radiology. J Vasc Interv Radiol. 1999; 10(4):491–8.

Bhat R, McBride K, Chakraverty S, Vikram R, Severn A. Primary cutting balloon angioplasty for treatment of venous stenoses in native hemodialysis fistulas: long-term results from three centers. Cardiovasc Intervent Radiol. 2007;30:1166–70.

Bittl JA. Venous rupture during percutaneous treatment of hemodialysis fistulas and grafts. Catheter Cardiovasc Interv. 2009;74(7):1097–101.

Chakraverty S, Meier MAJ, Aarts JCNM, Ross RA, Griffiths GD. Cutting-balloon-associated vascular rupture after failed standard balloon angioplasty. Cardiovasc Intervent Radiol. 2006;28:661–4.

Guiu B, Loffroy R, Ben Salem D, Cercueil JP, Aho S, Mousson C, Krausé D. Angioplasty of long venous stenosis in hemodialysis access: at last an indication for cutting balloon? J Vasc Interv Radiol. 2007;18(8): 994–1000.

Wu C-C, Lin M-C, Pu S-Y, Tsai K-C, Wen S-C. Comparison of cutting balloon versus high-pressure balloon angioplasty for resistant venous stenoses of native hemodialysis fistulas. J Vasc Interv Radiol. 2008; 19(6):877–83.

Chapter 32
Circumferential Balloon Rupture and Retained Fragments During Fistuloplasty and Thrombolysis of a Thrombosed Fistula

Robert P. Allison, Anna Maria Belli, Joo-Young Chun, Raymond Chung, Raj Das, Andrew England, Karen Flood, Marie-France Giroux, Richard G. McWilliams, Robert Morgan, Nik Papadakos, Jai V. Patel, Raf Patel, Uday Patel, Lakshmi Ratnam, Reddi Prasad Yadavali, and John Rose

Abstract This case illustrates management of a thrombosed dialysis fistula. During this process an angioplasty balloon ruptured circumferentially leaving part of the balloon within the fistula. Successful retrieval of the balloon fragment is outlined.

Keywords Thrombosed fistula • Balloon angioplasty • Complications • Balloon rupture • Fragment retrieval

---

R.P. Allison
Department of Interventional Radiology, University Hospitals Southampton, Southampton, Hampshire, UK

A.M. Belli
Department of Radiology, St. George's Hospital and Medical School, Blackshaw Road, London SW17 0RE, UK
e-mail: anna.belli@stgeorges.nhs.uk

J.-Y. Chun • R. Chung • R. Das • R. Morgan • N. Papadakos
Department of Radiology, St. George's Hospital,
London, UK

A. England
Department of Radiography, University of Salford, Manchester, UK

K. Flood
Department of Vascular Radiology,
Leeds General Infirmary, Leeds, UK

M.-F. Giroux
Department of Radiology, CHUM-Centre Hospitalier
de l'Université de Montréal, Montreal, QC, Canada

R.G. McWilliams
Department of Radiology, Royal Liverpool
University Hospital, Liverpool, UK

J.V. Patel
Department of Radiology, The Leeds Teaching
Hospitals NHS Trust, Leeds, West Yorkshire, UK

R. Patel
Department of Radiology,
The Leeds Teaching Hospitals NHS Trust,
Leeds, West Yorkshire, UK
e-mail: rafpatel@gmail.com

U. Patel
Department of Diagnostic Radiology, St. George's Hospital and
Medical School, Blackshaw Road, SW17 0QT London, UK
e-mail: uday.patel@stgeorges.nhs.uk

L. Ratnam
Department of Radiology, St. George's Hospital,
Blackshaw Road, SW17 0QT London, UK
e-mail: lakshmi.ratnam@nhs.net

R.P. Yadavali
Department of Radiology, Aberdeen Royal
Infirmary, Aberdeen, UK

J. Rose
Department of Interventional Radiology,
Freeman Hospital, Newcastle Upon Tyne
Hospitals NHS Trust, Newcastle upon Tyne, UK

Case History

A 45-year-old man presented with low flow velocity and clot formation during dialysis through a long-standing left brachiocephalic fistula. An ultrasound examination demonstrated occlusive thrombus at the level of the arterial anastomosis extending into the fistula. He attended the interventional radiology unit for attempted salvage of the fistula.

Procedure

A micropunture set was used to gain retrograde access of the fistula, and a 4 Fr vascular sheath was inserted. A hydrophilic wire and Cobra catheter were used to cross the occlusive thrombus, which was confirmed on fistulography. Bolus doses (total 15 mg) of recombinant tissue plasminogen activator (rTPA) were given directly into the thrombus followed by balloon maceration of the thrombus, using a 6 × 40 mm low-profile balloon inflated at low pressure. A waist was seen during this time, indicating an underlying juxta-anastomotic fistula stenosis as the cause of thrombosis.

The 4 Fr sheath was upsized to 6 Fr and the wire exchanged for a 0.018″ platinum-tipped wire to allow a 4-mm-diameter cutting balloon to be used, followed by a 6 × 40 mm low-profile balloon. Successful de-waisting of the balloon was seen; however, an audible "pop" was heard during inflation, suggestive of balloon rupture. On attempted removal it was noted that the balloon markers were separating apart, as if the balloon was stretching (Fig. 32.1). A diagnosis of circumferential balloon rupture, with retained distal fragment, was made.

The proximal balloon fragment and delivery system were easily removed, leaving the distal balloon fragment still on the platinum plus wire. To remove the distal fragment, a vascular snare (loop-shaped snare) was inserted over the platinum plus wire and through the 6 Fr sheath. The distal end of the wire was successfully snared and when both the wire and snare were retracted, the balloon fragment was pulled into and through

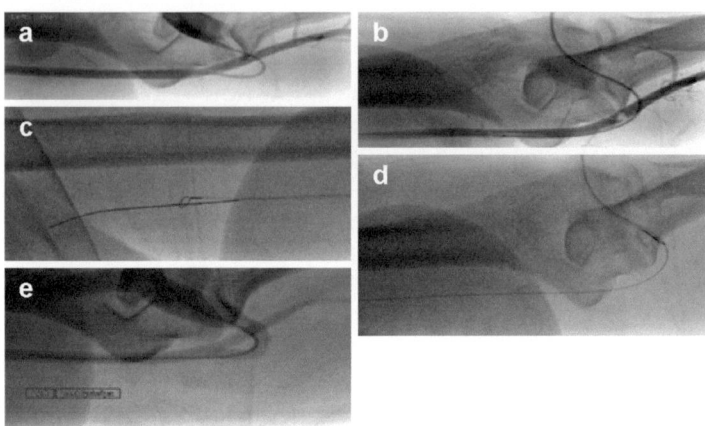

FIGURE 32.1 (**a**) shows contrast seen filling the brachial artery and the proximal fistula. (**b**) was taken after removal of the cutting balloon (see text). The distal balloon marker is seen, but the proximal marker is not on image. To remove the retained balloon fragment, the platinum plus wire was snared using a loop snare (**c**), entrapping the distal balloon fragment, and this is seen being removed (**d**). (**e**) shows good flow within the fistula, with no residual thrombus or balloon fragments

the 6 Fr vascular sheath. Check angiography confirmed that there were no residual fragments and good fistula flow.

Discussion

Overdistension and balloon rupture may occur when excessive inflation pressure is applied. Angioplasty balloons are rated according to a "nominal," "rated burst pressure." and "burst pressure." Nominal pressure is that pressure at which the balloon reaches its nominal diameter, whereas the rated burst pressure is that pressure to which the balloon can be inflated with a negligible risk of bursting (manufacturers test their balloons to a 95 % confidence limit that 99 % of their balloons will not burst at the rated burst pressure). Burst pressure is the average pressure required to rupture a

Chapter 32. Retained Fragments Post Balloon Rupture

balloon. From this it is clear that extreme care is required when the pressures exceed the rated burst pressure.

Balloon rupture is more frequent in stents (e.g., balloon-mounted stents), tight stenoses, and if the rated burst pressure is exceeded. It is also more common after multiple distensions. Rupture of modern balloon usually results in a longitudinal linear tear, without fragmentation and can be easily removed as a single entity. Less than 1 % of balloons will tear circumferentially. If this happens, there is a problem in withdrawing the balloon back through the sheath as the balloon tends to crumple and block the sheath – in a similar fashion to walking backwards through a doorway with an open umbrella.

In this case, the distal balloon fragment remained on the platinum plus wire, making snaring with a loop-shaped snare and retrieval possible. However, if the distal fragment of balloon becomes free-floating, techniques using a basket snare or careful use of retrieval forceps could be employed to remove the fragment.

If endovascular techniques are unsuccessful, then surgical removal is necessary to prevent migration into the brachial artery, resulting in distal limb ischemia, or re-thrombosis of the fistula if it remains in the venous outflow.

Tips

- Collateral veins can be used to access a fistula without having to directly puncture the fistula.
- The burst pressure should not be exceeded during balloon inflation.
- Circumferential balloon rupture is very rare; however, if it occurs, attempts at purely pulling the balloon back through the sheath are likely to be unsuccessful.
- If the balloon remains on the wire, vascular snares can be used to snare the wire and collapse the balloon fragment in order to pull this back through the sheath.
- Free-floating balloon fragments can be caught and retrieved using basket snares.

Commentary

Snares can be a simple loop in shape or more complex "basket"-like devices.

When used to grasp a free-floating fragment, the loop snare is inserted through its own cannula. When the snare exits from the tip of the cannula, it assumes its predetermined round loop shape. This is used to encircle any free end of the fragment, and when the cannula is advanced over the snare, the loop will tighten around and firmly grasp the fragment. Once grasped, the cannula and snare are removed as single unit with the caught fragment.

If, however, the fragment is not free-floating but still on a guidewire wire, then the loop snare can be used coaxially as shown in this case. The external end of the guidewire is threaded through the loop, and the snare is advanced coaxially over the guidewire and subsequently around the fragment. Once the snare loop is closed tightly, the fragment can be pulled into the sheath over the guidewire.

Thus, the essentials necessary for this maneuver are that a suitably large vascular sheath is in place such that it will accommodate the coaxial insertion of the snare mechanism and a guidewire and also accommodate the fragment. If necessary, the sheath should be upsized before the attempted snaring. Entry of the fragment into the sheath is easier if it has been grasped near its tip rather than in the center. Occasionally, the fragment will not fully enter into the sheath, but if the practitioner can be confident that it is firmly wedged in the vascular sheath, then the sheath and fragment can be retrieved together, but with great care and under constant fluoroscopic vision.

Finally, it should be ensured that all the fragments have been successfully removed at the end of the procedure. With radiopaque objects this is straightforward. With lucent fragments, check angiography may be sufficient. If this is not feasible, ultrasound should be considered. Alternatively, the retrieved pieces should be lined up to confirm that the broken ends match perfectly without any gaps.

Further Reading

Nukta E, Meier B, Urban P, Muller T. Circumferential rupture and entrapment of a balloon-on-a-wire device during coronary angioplasty. Cathet Cardiovasc Diagn. 1990;20(2):123–5.

Selby JB, Oliva VL, Tegtmeyer CJ. Circumferential rupture of an angioplasty balloon with detachment from the shaft: case report. Cardiovasc Intervent Radiol. 1992;15(2):113–6.

Vanmaele RG, D'Archambeau OC, Van Schil PE, Van Landuyt KA, De Schepper AM. Ruptured balloon separation during percutaneous transluminal renal artery angioplasty. Eur J Vasc Surg. 1993;7(1):104–6.

Yune HY, Klatte EC. Circumferential tear of percutaneous transluminal angioplasty catheter balloon. AJR Am J Roentgenol. 1980;135:395–6.

Chapter 33
Hemorrhage After Transjugular Liver Biopsy

Robert P. Allison, Anna Maria Belli, Joo-Young Chun, Raymond Chung, Raj Das, Andrew England, Karen Flood, Marie-France Giroux, Richard G. McWilliams, Robert Morgan, Nik Papadakos, Jai V. Patel, Raf Patel, Uday Patel, Lakshmi Ratnam, Reddi Prasad Yadavali, and John Rose

Abstract This case describes hemorrhage following transjugular liver biopsy in a cirrhotic patient. Various tips are given with respect to technical approach and steps which can be taken to minimize the risk of such a complication.

Keywords Transjugular liver biopsy • Complications • Hemorrhage • Embolization

---

R.P. Allison
Department of Interventional Radiology,
University Hospitals Southampton,
Southampton, Hampshire, UK

A.M. Belli
Department of Radiology, St. George's Hospital
and Medical School, Blackshaw Road,
London SW17 0RE, UK
e-mail: anna.belli@stgeorges.nhs.uk

J.-Y. Chun • R. Chung • R. Das • R. Morgan • N. Papadakos
Department of Radiology, St. George's Hospital, London, UK

A. England
Department of Radiography, University of Salford, Manchester, UK

K. Flood
Department of Vascular Radiology,
Leeds General Infirmary, Leeds, UK

M.-F. Giroux
Department of Radiology,
CHUM-Centre Hospitalier de l'Université de Montréal,
Montreal, QC, Canada

R.G. McWilliams
Department of Radiology, Royal Liverpool University Hospital,
Liverpool, UK

J.V. Patel
Department of Radiology, The Leeds Teaching
Hospitals NHS Trust, Leeds, West Yorkshire, UK

R. Patel
Department of Radiology,
The Leeds Teaching Hospitals NHS Trust,
Leeds, West Yorkshire, UK
e-mail: rafpatel@gmail.com

U. Patel
Department of Diagnostic Radiology,
St. George's Hospital and Medical School,
Blackshaw Road, SW17 0QT London, UK
e-mail: uday.patel@stgeorges.nhs.uk

L. Ratnam
Department of Radiology, St. George's Hospital,
Blackshaw Road, SW17 0QT London, UK
e-mail: lakshmi.ratnam@nhs.net

R.P. Yadavali
Department of Radiology, Aberdeen Royal
Infirmary, Aberdeen, UK

J. Rose
Department of Interventional Radiology,
Freeman Hospital, Newcastle Upon Tyne
Hospitals NHS Trust, Newcastle upon Tyne, UK

Case History

A 46-year-old man with a known history of excess alcohol intake presented with acute decompensated liver failure with ascites, jaundice, and coagulopathy. The patient was referred for transjugular liver biopsy (TJLB) and tunnelled ascitic drain placement. Pre-procedural blood tests showed raised bilirubin (230), low hemoglobin (8.5), low platelet count (80), and raised INR (2.0). Therefore, packed red cells, vitamin K, and fresh frozen plasma were given prior to the procedure.

Procedure

A tunnelled ascitic line was first placed under US guidance for large-volume ascites. One liter of straw-colored fluid was drained. Transjugular liver biopsy (TJLB) was then performed from a right internal jugular vein approach. The right hepatic vein was selectively catheterized with a multipurpose catheter. The catheter was then removed, and a long sheath advanced into the hepatic vein over a stiff guidewire. A biopsy needle was inserted via the sheath into the hepatic vein, and four 19 G core biopsies were taken with the sheath tip directed anteriorly (Fig. 33.1a). Post biopsy venogram showed no evidence of contrast extravasation. The patient was hemodynamically stable during and immediately following the procedure and was transferred back to the ward.

Six hours following the procedure, bloody ascitic fluid was drained from the abdominal drain, and the patient became hemodynamically unstable. Post biopsy bleeding was suspected, and urgent CT angiogram with view to embolization was advised. The patient was deemed too unstable for transfer by the clinical team. Repeat bloods showed a significant drop in Hb (5.1), low platelet count (53), and elevated INR (2.4). CT was delayed while the patient was fluid resuscitated, and attempts were made to correct coagulopathy with various blood products. The patient required anaesthetic support

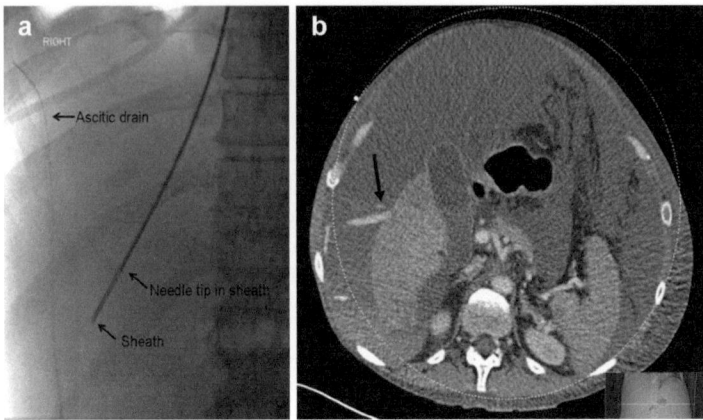

FIGURE 33.1 (**a**) Position of the vascular sheath and biopsy needle prior to biopsy. The sheath was retracted approx 1 cm from this position prior to each biopsy with a 2 cm throw. (**b**) Post biopsy, CT angiogram shows a markedly shrunken liver and active contrast extravasation (*arrow*) from the liver capsule

and intubation prior to transfer to radiology 5 h later. CT angiogram showed a markedly shrunken cirrhotic liver with active bleeding from the liver capsule (Fig. 33.1b).

The patient was transferred immediately to the interventional radiology suite. During the femoral arterial puncture, it was noted that there was little pulsatility and the arterial blood appeared pink and diluted. A selective right hepatic angiogram confirmed active contrast extravasation from a capsular branch (Fig. 33.2a). The right hepatic artery was embolized with gelatin sponge with successful occlusion of the bleeding vessel on angiography (Fig. 33.2b). However, the patient remained unstable throughout the procedure, and it was evident the patient had developed disseminated intravascular coagulopathy (DIC). Despite supportive measures in the ICU, the patient died a few hours later.

Discussion

Liver biopsy is the most specific test to assess the nature and severity of liver disease. TJLB is performed when percutaneous biopsy is contraindicated due to coagulopathy, ascites,

Chapter 33. Hemorrhage After Transjugular Liver Biopsy 255

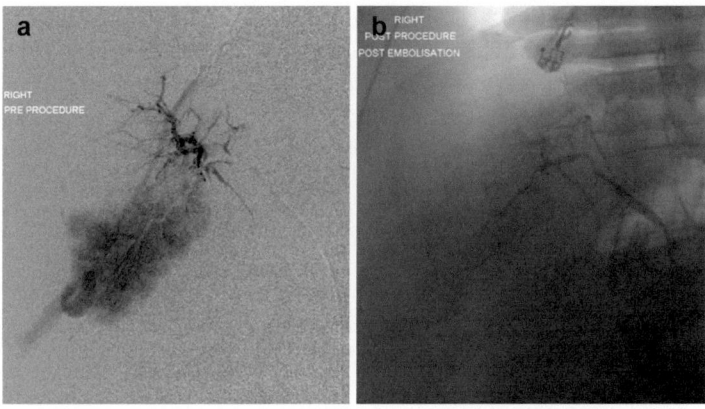

FIGURE 33.2 (**a**) Selective right hepatic angiogram shows active contrast extravasation from a capsular branch. (**b**) Right hepatic angiogram following embolization with gelatin sponge shows successful occlusion of the bleeding capsular vessel

and liver transplantation. The technique minimizes the risk of bleeding as the liver tissue is obtained from within the vascular system and avoids breaching the liver capsule. It is important to avoid peripheral positioning of the biopsy needle as the liver capsule can be perforated when the needle is advanced through the wall of the hepatic vein.

TJLB is a safe procedure with a low major complication rate (0.6 %) and mortality rate (0.09 %), considering that it is performed in patients with coagulopathy. Complication rates are significantly higher in smaller livers which increase the technical difficulty and risk of capsular perforation.

This patient was unsuitable for percutaneous biopsy due to coagulopathy and gross ascites. Although measures were taken to correct the underlying coagulopathy prior to the procedure, the complication occurred due to inadvertent breach of the liver capsule by the biopsy needle. This could have been avoided if the degree of fibrosis and size of the liver were known prior to the procedure and extra care was taken to obtain the biopsies more centrally.

In addition to the technical error, there was a significant delay between the time the complication was identified and embolization of the bleeding vessel. Resuscitation and reversal of coagulopathy are necessary components to managing patients in acute hemorrhagic shock. However, these supportive measures are not effective if the bleeding source is not controlled. It is also important to note that once the patient develops DIC due to prolonged blood loss, embolization becomes less effective and is associated with significantly poorer outcomes.

Tips

- Perform on table US prior to TJLB to confirm liver size and approximate the liver edge.
- Confirm the right hepatic vein has been catheterized with lateral fluoroscopy – the right hepatic vein courses posteriorly in the liver.
- Perform hepatic venography prior to biopsy to evaluate the anatomy and the sheath tip position.
- Perform a post biopsy venogram to look for extravasation from capsular breach.
- Do not delay imaging and embolization in unstable bleeding patients. Stabilization of an acutely bleeding patient can only be achieved if the source of hemorrhage is controlled.

Commentary

Transjugular liver biopsy is often performed in patients with a high risk of hemorrhage due to abnormal clotting, and meticulous technique is helpful in reducing complication rates. After catheterization of the hepatic vein, fluoroscopy in a true lateral position should be performed to confirm the catheter is posteriorly placed within the liver – the catheter should be seen to be adjacent to the patient's spine. Thus, when the sheath is pointed anteriorly (using arrow on the sheath hub of transjugular biopsy set), the biopsy needle will shoot out into the maximal amount of liver parenchyma. Following each pass of

Chapter 33. Hemorrhage After Transjugular Liver Biopsy 257

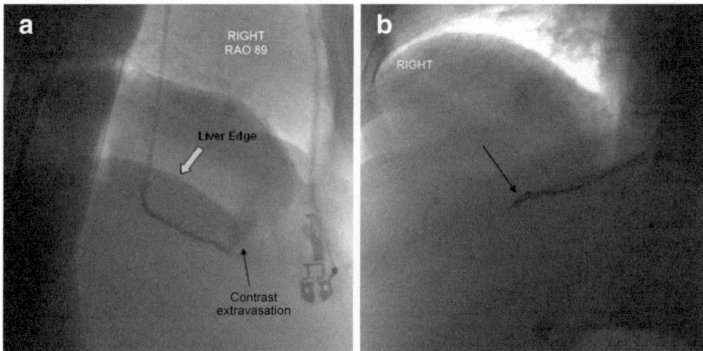

FIGURE 33.3 (**a**) Post biopsy injection in another cirrhotic patient shows active contrast extravasation into the ascites surrounding the liver. (**b**) A 5 mm fibered coil (*black arrow*) was deployed immediately through the catheter, post coil venogram shows backfilling of the hepatic vein only with no contrast extravasation. The patient remained stable throughout

the biopsy needle, contrast injection should be performed to check for capsular breach or arterial injury. If this is identified at the time when the sheath is in position, a fibered coil can be deployed directly from the position in which the venogram is performed in order to stop any bleeding (Fig. 33.3a, b). Prompt treatment will often avert adverse consequences.

A risk assessment should also be performed in those patients who are felt to be particularly technically challenging. Although tissue diagnosis can be useful in confirming a diagnosis, in situations where this is unlikely to result in a change in the patient's management, it may be more appropriate not to proceed.

Further Reading

Bravo AA, Sheth SG, Chopra S. Liver biopsy. N Engl J Med. 2001; 344(7):495–500.

Kalambokis G, Manousou P, Vibhakorn S, Marelli L, Cholongitas E, Senzolo M, Patch D, Burroughs AK. Transjugular liver biopsy – indications, adequacy, quality of specimens, and complications – a systematic review. J Hepatol. 2007;47:284–94.

Index

A
Abdominal aortic aneurysm (AAA)
  bifurcated stent graft, 151
  conical aortic neck, 141
  and FEVAR, 131
  Gore bifurcated device, 123
Abscess
  biliary sepsis/ischemia, 196
  formation, 194–195
  hepatic artery embolization, 194
  inflammatory markers, 193
  residual collection, 193
Angioplasty balloon
  application, 18, 23
  balloon-assisted technique, 218
  cephalad and caudal approaches, 208
  inflation, 85, 86, 125
  nominal pressure, 246
  recommended pressures, 60
  reinflation, 88
  right femoral approach, 85
  stent graft, 86
  Terumo guide wire and Cobra 2 catheter, 86
  venogram postprimary cutting, 238, 239
Anticoagulation, 223, 230
Aortic neck
  dilatation, 118
  and endograft, 120
  fabric markers, 115, 116
  open repair and surgical banding, 118
  Palmaz stent, 118
  thrombus-lined, 118
Arterial dissection
  balloon-expanded stent, 72, 73
  blood flow, 73
  CIA and EIA stenoses, 71
  common iliac artery, 71–72
  contralateral groin, 73
  flow-limiting dissections/elastic recoil, 72
  4 Fr sheath, 72
  MRA, 71
  self-expanding stent, 72
  stenting, 72
Arterial stenting. *See* Iatrogenic iliac artery rupture

Arteriography, 31, 32
Arterioportal fistula and liver hemorrhage
  angiography, 201–202
  femoral artery approach, 201
  NASH, 201
  TACE, 202–203
  tract ablation, 203–204
  tumor, right liver lobe, 204
Arteriovenous fistulae (AVF), 14, 15, 17

B

Balloon angioplasty, 223–224
Balloon-assisted technique, 218, 230
Balloon-expandable stent, 91, 92, 93, 143, 144, 145
Balloon rupture and retained fragments
  angiography, 245–246
  brachial artery, 248
  brachiocephalic fistula, 245
  collateral veins, 247
  endovascular techniques, 246
  proximal balloon fragment and delivery system, 245
  and rtPA, 245
Bowel perforation
  biochemical markers, renal function, 178
  complications, 179
  distal ureteric stricture, 177
  exploratory laparotomy, 178
  interpolar calyx, transplant kidney, 177
  lower pole calyx, 180
  and PCN, 180
  peritonitis/bowel obstruction, 181
  post-nephrostomy insertion nephrostogram, 177
  renal function and hydronephrosis, 177
  small bowel injury, 179
  visceral injury, 178

C

"Catheter-snare technique", 230, 231
Central venous catheter (CVC)
  angioplasty balloons, 26
  arteriography, 31
  arteriovenous, 23
  brachiocephalic vein and SVC, 31–32
  Dialock port, 24
  endovascular techniques, 25–26
  12F sheath, 23
  gooseneck snare, 23
  hemodialysis, 31
  hemothorax, 33
  right atrium, 23
  thorax, 32
  venogram, 34–35
  venous access ports, 25
  venous injury, 32
CEUS. *See* Contrast-enhanced ultrasound (CEUS)
CFA. *See* Common femoral artery (CFA)
CFV. *See* Common femoral vein (CFV)
CIV. *See* Common iliac vein (CIV)
CL. *See* Contralateral limb (CL)
Cobra catheter, 71, 79, 245
Coil displacement, 124, 125
Coil retrieval, 4
Color Doppler ultrasound, 40, 42

Common femoral artery (CFA), 65, 73
Common femoral vein (CFV), 9, 10
Common hepatic artery
  active hemorrhage, 102
  angiography, 99, 100
  angioplasty balloon, 103
  coaxial microcatheter, 99
  Cobra and Berenstein catheters, 99
  coil embolization/occlusion, 102
  and CTA, 102
  deployment, 101
  endovascular treatment, 100
  extravasation and pseudoaneurysm, 100
  and GDA, 99
  malposition, 101
  microcatheter wire and catheter, 101
  portal vein, 102
  right HA, 99
  stent grafts, 102–103
Common iliac vein (CIV), 109
Complications
  bowel perforation, transplant nephrostomy, 179
  brachiocephalic vein, 111
  catastrophic, 87
  common iliac artery, 128
  hepatic artery, 80–81
  iliac angioplasty and stenting, 86
  life-threatening, 87
  pigtail aortogram, 78
  proximal type 1 endoleaks, 119
  stent detachment, 93
Contralateral limb (CL)
  aortic endograft, 155
  brachial artery, 154
  maldeployment, 155
  pre-procedural imaging, 154
Contrast-enhanced ultrasound (CEUS), 123
Contrast-related nephropathy, 186
CT angiography (CTA), 102

D

Deep vein thrombus (DVT), 229
DIC. *See* Disseminated intravascular coagulopathy (DIC)
Displaced coil, 4
Dissection
  and SMA
    patent lumen, 79
    pigtail catheter, 78
    post-stent deployment, 80
    Sos Omni catheter, 78
    Terumo wire, 79
  spasm and minor dissection, hepatic artery, 80–81
  and TACE, 81
Disseminated intravascular coagulopathy (DIC), 254, 256
Distal embolization
  angiography, 65
  catheters, 67
  and CFA, 65
  clot aspiration, 67
  limb, 67
  post-angioplasty, 65
  and SFA, 65
  thromboaspiration, 66
  thrombus, PT, 66

Doppler ultrasound
  aneurysm and endoleak, 123
  left iliac limb and posterior wall, 123
DVT. *See* Deep vein thrombus (DVT)

E
EIA. *See* External iliac artery (EIA)
Embolization
  chemoembolization, 80–81
  coil protruding, 3, 4
  and CXR, 194
  displaced coil, 4
  "dropped", 4
  hepatic artery, 194
  interventional radiology, 3
  microcatheter, 82
  NET metastases, 195
  and PES (*see* Post-embolization syndrome (PES))
  right renal, 169
  sheath, 4
  and TACE (*see* Transarterial chemoembolization (TACE))
  transarterial and translumbar, 135
  transcatheter, 170
  tumor necrosis, 196
Endovascular aortic aneurysm repair (EVAR)
  aortic neck, 143
  and aorto-uniiliac (AUI), 154
  button-mushroom, 153, 154
  catheter, 152
  and CL, 155
  embolization coils, 152
  endovascular solution, 153, 154
  fenestrated cuff, 118
  internal and external iliac artery, 151, 152
  maldeployment (*see* Maldeployed limb)
  open aortic surgery, 161
  Palmaz stent, 152, 153
  post-deployment angiography, 152
  proximal type 1 endoleaks, 117, 119, 127
  radio-opaque markers, 155
  stent-graft design and aneurysm morphology, 153
  type 4 thoracoabdominal aneurysm, 159
  Zenith bifurcated device, 141
Endovascular techniques, 25–26, 246
EVAR. *See* Endovascular aortic aneurysm repair (EVAR)
External iliac artery (EIA)
  angiography, 71
  digital subtraction angiogram, 92
  occlusion, 91, 92
  patient's symptoms, 91

F
Femoral artery pseudoaneurysm
  balloon inflation, 42
  chest pain, 39
  descending artery, 39
  Doppler ultrasound, 40
  hallux, 40

iatrogenic
  pseudoaneurysms, 41
 peripheral pulses, 40
 ST-elevation myocardial
  infarction, 39
 thrombin injection, 41
 treatment options, 41
Fenestrated cuff, 118, 120
Fenestrated endovascular
  aortic aneurysm
  repair (FEVAR), 131
Fistula rupture
  post-fistuloplasty
  arterial anastomosis, 237
 cutting balloons, 239
 dialysis fistulas, 237–238
 fistulogram, 237
 stenosis, 237
 stenting, 239
 thrombosis and vessel
  rupture, 240
Foreign body retrieval
 catheter, 9
 and CFV, 9, 10
 coaxial snare
  technique, 11
 interventional radiology, 9
 and IVC, 11
 loop snares/goose neck
  snares, 10
 novel techniques, 9
 snares, 11
 vascular sheath, 9, 10

G

Gastroduodenal artery (GDA)
 coeliac/hepatic arteries,
  99, 101
 coil embolization, 99
GDA. *See* Gastroduodenal
  artery (GDA)

H

HA. *See* Hepatic artery (HA)
HCC. *See* Hepatocellular
  carcinoma (HCC)
Hemorrhage. *See also*
  Nephrostomy
 angiograms, 169
 angiography, 171
 blood hemoglobin
  level, 171
 Brödel's line, 171
 catheter, 171
 CT images, 172
 hydronephrosis and
  hydroureter, 169
 minor hematuria, 170
 nephrostomy insertion, 170
 renal artery (*see* Renal
  arterial hemorrhage)
 vascular injury, 170
Hepatic artery
 isolation, 77
 replacement, 77
 and RHA, 77
 spasm and minor
  dissections, 80–81
Hepatic artery (HA),
  99, 100, 101
Hepatocellular carcinoma
 (HCC), 77, 201, 202

I

Iatrogenic iliac artery rupture
 Amplatz guide wire, 86
 angioplasty balloon, 85, 86
 balloon expandable/
  self-expanding stent
  graft, 87
 emergency bypass surgery, 88
 external iliac artery, 87
 left external iliac artery, 85

Iatrogenic iliac artery rupture (*cont.*)
  life-threatening complication, 86, 87
  management, 87
  recanalization, 88
  reinflation, 88
  retrograde ipsilateral stenting, 88
  right femoral approach, 85
  Terumo guide wire, 86
  vascular interventional radiologists, 88
Iliac angioplasty, 88, 91, 94
Iliac artery
  angiography, 71
  angioplasty, 73
  chronic, 72
  common, 71–72
  and EIA, 71
Inferior mesenteric artery (IMA)
  aneurysm, 131, 132
  left colic, sigmoid and superior rectal branches, 133
  microcatheter, 132
  type 2 endoleak, 136
  visualization, 136
  Vortex coils, 133
Inferior vena cava (IVC) filter
  anticoagulation, 230
  balloon-assisted technique, 218
  balloon dilatation, 210
  "branch technique", 230
  catheter removal, 216
  "catheter-snare technique", 230
  cavogram, 216
  conventional techniques, 218
  DVT, 229
  femoral and jugular approaches, 217, 229
  loop-snare technique, 217, 218
  maneuvers, 208, 209
  optional filters, 210
  portal venous phase, 207
  procedure, 208
  pulmonary emboli, 229
  renal vein, 231
  retrieval (*see* Retrieval, IVC filter)
  thrombosis and pulmonary embolism, 215, 229
  tilting, 208–209
  twist technique, 218
  vena cava tributaries, 232
  venogram, 216
IVC filter. *See* Inferior vena cava (IVC) filter

L
Laser-assisted sheath technique, 225
Loop-snare technique, 216, 217, 218

M
Magnetic resonance angiography (MRA), 65, 71, 91
Maldeployed limb, 151, 153, 155
Migrated stent graft
  angioplasty balloon, 107
  arterial/venous system, 109–110
  balloon inflation, 107, 109
  bare-metal stents, 110
  "catching", 110

and CIV, 109
guide wire, 109
hand-crimped balloon-expandable stents, 111
right brachiocephalic vein, 107, 108
"salvaging", 110
snare, 110
and SVC, 107, 108
and TIPS, 107, 108
venography, 107
Modular disconnection
anatomical changes, 161
bridging endograft, 165
type 3 endoleak, 161
Vanguard stent graft, 163
MRA. *See* Magnetic resonance angiography (MRA)

N
NASH. *See* Nonalcoholic steatohepatitis (NASH)
n-Butyl cyanoacrylate (n-BCA), 119
Nephrostomy
arterial phase CT, 169
balloon dilation catheter, 170
hemorrhagic complications, 170
perirenal and retroperitoneal hemorrhage, 170
posterior-facing calyx, 170
Neuroendocrine tumor (NET)
embolization, 193
metastases, 195
neoplasm, 195
Nonalcoholic steatohepatitis (NASH), 201

P
Percutaneous nephrostomy tube (PCN), 177, 180
Post-angioplasty, 72
Post-embolization syndrome (PES), 196, 197
Pressure inflation device, 60
Proximal cuff
impinging, 117
implantation and molds, 115, 116
insertion, 118
Pyrexia, tumor embolization
abscess (*see* Abscess)
angiography demonstration, 193
blood parameters, 196
CT scan, 193
CXR, 193, 194
embolic particles, 195
5 Fr vascular sheath, 193
hepatic artery embolization, 195
intercostal approach, 193
metastasis, 194
NET liver metastases, 195
pogenic abscess, 194
prophylactic antibiotics, 197
and PVA, 195
residual collection, 194
tumor necrosis and drains, 195

R
Recombinant tissue plasminogen activator (rtPA), 47–48, 50, 51, 245

Renal arterial hemorrhage
    bilateral femoral punctures, 185
    elective left renal artery stenting, 185
    hemodynamic instability, 187
    immediate repeat angiography, 185
    left stenosis, 189
    normal perfusion pressure theory, 186
    pathophysiological mechanisms, 186
    renal bleeding, 188
    risk factors, 187
Renal artery occlusion
    and AAA, 141
    anchor stent, 142
    balloon-expandable stent, 143, 144
    bare suprarenal stent struts, 144, 146
    catheterization and manipulation, 147
    caudal traction, 144
    contralateral groin, 145
    coronal CT reformatted image and angiogram, 141
    and EVAR, 141
    intra operative aortogram, 144–145
    ostia, 143
    projectional errors, 146
    reversed curve catheter, 141, 142
    sheath, 142, 143
    stent graft, 144
    stent struts and left renal artery, 142–143
    surgical extra-anatomical revascularization, 146

Renal artery thrombosis, 186
Retrieval, IVC filter
    anticoagulation, 223
    balloon angioplasty, 223–224
    cavogram, 223
    factors, filter incorporation, 224
    laser-assisted sheath technique, 225
    neovascularization, 225–226
    stenosis and clot formation, 225
Right hepatic artery (RHA)
    chemoembolization, 80
    embolization, 254
    microcatheter wire and catheter, 101
    Sidewinder catheter, 77
    Sos Omni catheter, 77
    stent graft, 101
rtPA. *See* Recombinant tissue plasminogen activator (rtPA)
Rupture
    arterial, 86, 87
    iliac artery (*see* Iatrogenic iliac artery rupture)
    left external iliac artery, 85

S

Sidewinder catheter, 77
SMA. *See* Superior mesenteric artery (SMA)
Snare
    femoral vein, 108
    guidewire, 9
    intravascular objects retrieval, 10
    size and location, 11
    stent, proximal end, 110

Sos Omni catheter, 77, 78, 81
Stent
  atrium, 159
  hemostasis post deployment, 238
  renal artery branch, 160
  venous rupture, 239
Stent detachment
  balloon-mounted stent detaches, 93, 94
  bilateral iliac angioplasty, 91
  common iliac stenoses, 91
  detached balloon-mounted stent, 91, 92
  digital subtraction angiogram, 91, 92
  disastrous complication, 93
  6-Fr retrograde right CFA puncture, 91
  guide catheter and sheath, 93
  ipsilateral access, 94
  management, 93
  patient's symptoms, 91
  right CIA/EIA, 91, 92
  snare, 93
Stent graft
  angioplasty balloon, 103
  balloon-expandable, 86, 99
  balloon-mounted, 102–103
  deployment, 101, 102
  maldeployment, 103
  management, 87
  right and left HA, 99, 101
  self-expanding, 87
Stenting
  adjacent/buttressing, 102
  balloon-expanded, 72, 73
  and CIA, 71
  flow-limiting dissection, 72
  iliac angioplasty, 94
  primary, 72
  secondary, 72
  self-expanding, 72, 92
Stent malposition, 101, 103
Stiff guide wire, 80
Superficial femoral artery (SFA)
  angioplasty
    balloon reinflation, 57–58
    extravasation, 59
    pressure inflation device, 60
    prosthetic aortic valve, 57
    recanalization, 57
    thorax/abdomen, 58
    vessel rupture, 59
  thrombosis post-angioplasty
    distal embolization, 51
    luminal wire position, 48
    and rtPA, 47
    stenting, 51
    thromboaspiration, 49, 51, 66
Superior mesenteric artery (SMA)
  dissection (*see* Dissection)
  and RHA, 77, 80, 81
  type 2 endoleak, 132
Superior vena cava (SVC)
  Amplatz Gooseneck snare, 16
  and AVF, 14
  balloon inflated within stent graft, 109
  cardiac chambers and pulmonary arterial, 18–19
  indications, 17–18
  migrated stent graft, 107, 108
  migration, 19
  restenosis and thrombosis, 18
  retrieval technique, 18

Superior vena cava (SVC) (*cont.*)
  stenosis, 14–15
  subclavian vein, 15
  symptoms, 17
  venoplast, 17
SVC. *See* Superior vena cava (SVC)

T

TACE. *See* Transarterial chemoembolization (TACE)
Terumo hydrophilic guide wire, 77, 79
Thromboaspiration, 51
TIPS. *See* Transjugular intrahepatic portosystemic shunt (TIPS)
TJLB. *See* Transjugular liver biopsy (TJLB)
Transarterial chemoembolization (TACE)
  acute dissection, 82
  Amplatz wire, 80
  antispasmodics, 80–81
  arterial dissection, 81–82
  arterioportal fistula, 203
  bare-metal stent, 82
  brachial artery access, 81
  Cobra catheter, 79
  complication, 78
  fetoprotein, 77
  fine caliber wires, 81
  HCC treatment, 77
  hepatitis C, 77
  hepatocellular carcinoma, 77
  modern small vessel catheters, 81
  patient, 80
  and RHA, 77
  semi-selective angiography, 81
  Sidewinder catheter, 77
  and SMA, 77
  soft-tipped guide wire, 77
  Sos Omni catheter, 77–78
  Terumo wire, 79
Transjugular intrahepatic portosystemic shunt (TIPS)
  primary intervention, 110
  right portal vein and hepatic vein, 107
Transjugular liver biopsy (TJLB)
  coagulopathy, 255–256
  complication rates, 255
  description, 253
  and DIC, 254
  femoral arterial puncture, 254
  hepatic venography, 256
  post biopsy injection, 256, 257
  vascular sheath, 253–254
Transplant nephrostomy, 179. *See also* Bowel perforation
Twist technique, 218
Type 1a endoleak
  aneurysm, 115
  aortic neck, 115, 118
  aortography, 115
  completion angiography, 117
  CT scan, 115
  deployment, 118
  embolic and thrombus-inducing agents, 119
  etiology, 119

and EVAR (*see*
Endovascular aortic
aneurysm repair
(EVAR))
fabric markers, 115
fenestrated cuffs, 120
fluoroscopic images, 115
follow-up catheter
aortogram, 115, 116
left renal artery ostium, 115
MIP image, 115, 116
n-BCA, 119
open aneurysm surgery,
118
Palmaz stent, 118
patients, 120
proximal cuff, 115, 117
secondary complication,
117
sizing problem, 118
stent-graft anchoring barb,
115
and type 2 endoleak, 119
Type 1b endoleak
buttock claudication
post-embolization,
127
and CEUS, 123
common iliac artery,
126–127
completion angiography,
125, 126
distal type 1 endoleak, 124
embolization coils, 124, 125
endurant iliac limb
extension, 124
EUROSTAR registry,
125–126
and EVAR (*see*
Endovascular aortic
aneurysm repair
(EVAR))
follow-up arterial phase, 123
Gore bifurcated device, 123
internal iliac arteries, 128
open aortic repair, 127
Palmaz stent, 127
patients, 125
stent-graft limbs,
124–125, 127
ultrasound-guided
puncture, 123
Type 1 endoleak, 123–124, 125,
126
Type 2 endoleak
angiogram, 134
catheter-based embolization
techniques, 136
CT scan, 131
and EVAR (*see*
Endovascular aortic
aneurysm repair
(EVAR))
and FEVAR, 131
identification, 115
and IMA, 131
inferior and superior
mesenteric
artery, 136
intrasac pressure
measurements, 135
microcatheter, 132
preoperative imaging, 136
pressurization, 119
and proximal type 1, 115
SMA angiogram, 132
transarterial and
translumbar
embolization, 135
Vortex coils, 132–134
Type 3 endoleak
abdominal radiographs,
162, 163
AneuRx device, 161, 164
branched endografts, 159,
161, 165

Type 3 endoleak (*cont.*)
    completion angiography, 160
    and EVAR (*see* Endovascular aortic aneurysm repair (EVAR))
    left iliac limb, 161, 162
    left renal stent and artery, 159
    modular disconnection, 161
    preliminary angiography, 160
    stent graft, 164

V
Venogram
    extravasation, 253, 256, 257
    IVC filter, 216
    postprimary cutting balloon angioplasty, 238
    right brachiocephalic vein, 23, 24
    TIPS, 107
Vessel rupture
    acute extravasation, 237
    angioplasty, 57–58
    peripheral circulation, 58
    standard balloon angioplasty, 239
    thrombosis, 240

Z
Zenith bifurcated device, 141

MIX
Papier aus verantwortungsvollen Quellen
Paper from responsible sources
FSC® C105338

If you have any concerns about our products,
you can contact us on
ProductSafety@springernature.com

In case Publisher is established outside the EU,
the EU authorized representative is:
**Springer Nature Customer Service Center GmbH
Europaplatz 3, 69115 Heidelberg, Germany**

Printed by Libri Plureos GmbH
in Hamburg, Germany